THE FIGHT AGAINST ALZHEIMER'S

'Dr Sen's commitment to the caring and compassionate handling of people afflicted with Alzheimer's is an outstanding feature of a doctor who stands tall amongst physicians serving mankind[...] In time, this book will be embraced as a Bible of understanding and hope.'

Victor Banerjee
Actor

'An erudite and practical guidebook, written by a man who is a scholar, physician and researcher. It will provide a template and path to navigate through troubled waters.'

Aaron Feingold
MD, Physician and Author,
Chief of Cardiology, John F. Kennedy Memorial Hospital

'A great hand of care for those trapped in a ruthless disease as also for those who stand by them. A unique step by step approach.'

Ronald Brenner
MD, Chief of Psychiatry, Catholic Health Lines Hospital

'This new book from Shuvendu Sen, MD, is another home run for this ingenious medical practitioner. A brilliant writer, he compliments his medical knowledge flawlessly.'

Oliver Tuthill
Hollywood Filmmaker and Music Composer

'Dr Shuvendu Sen brings the nuances of the "how"', the "why" and the '"what" of Alzheimer's disease into our drawing rooms with a simple yet scientific narrative. We are reminded of the gray clouds looming overhead as the ageing population progresses towards the tsunami of dementia.'

Lt Gen. Madhuri Kanitkar
PVSM AVSM VSM (Retd),
Vice Chancellor, Maharashtra University of Health Sciences

'This book will be an excellent practical guide for close as well as extended family members who are ultimately the caretakers and caregivers in India. The book will help them recognize the onset of dementia and Alzheimer's.'

Sanjay Bhatnagar
Former Business Head and General Manager,
Bennett Coleman & Company Ltd, Times Group

'A wonderful read that narrates the challenges and triumphs related to the Alzheimer's disease[...] It introduces important approaches for anyone dealing with Alzheimer's.'

Andrew Newberg
MD, Professor, Department of Integrative Medicine and
Nutritional Sciences, Research Director,
Marcus Institute of Integrative Health,

'A chance meeting with Dr Sen back in 2017 has evolved into a lifelong friendship in the last six years. He was instrumental in the process of my most special directorial venture till date, Abhijaan.
This book on Alzheimer's brings out the best in him, and combines two equally brilliant aspects—one as an outstanding medical practitioner, the other as a gifted and passionate writer.'

Parambrata Chatterjee
Actor

'Dr Sen has written another informative and ground breaking bestseller! This is a book that every specialist, and every person who has a friend or family member afflicted with Alzheimer's, should read.'

Tara Walker
Hollywood Actress and Social Activist

THE FIGHT AGAINST ALZHEIMER'S

How to Prevent, Cure, Care, and Find Hope

DR SHUVENDU SEN

Winner of the prestigious **Nautilus Award**

RUPA

Published by
Rupa Publications India Pvt. Ltd 2024
7/16, Ansari Road, Daryaganj
New Delhi 110002

Sales centres:
Bengaluru Chennai
Hyderabad Jaipur Kathmandu
Kolkata Mumbai Prayagraj

Photo credits: Shuvendu Sen, Creative Commons

P-ISBN: 978-93-90260-75-1
E-ISBN: 978-93-90260-77-5

First impression 2024

10 9 8 7 6 5 4 3 2 1

Printed in India

CONTENTS

PREFACE

'The mind is its own place, and in itself can make a heaven of hell, a hell of heaven.'

—John Milton, English poet

ALZHEIMER'S: AN ENDEMIC, A HOUSEHOLD DISEASE

Didun went missing one evening. Her panic-stricken family searched the streets of Calcutta (now Kolkata). When she was eventually found close to midnight on a dead-end street, she was undressed, exposed to the moonlight. She seemed frozen, suspended in time and space, swaying back and forth.

When she was brought home, she slipped into a completely different persona. Seeming to fade into oblivion, she was not able to identify the once familiar faces. Looking in the mirror, she could not recognize herself. Over the next few weeks, she could not carry out her basic chores.

I had been one of my grandmother's favourites. She had been hell-bent on making me a poet. But she then spent her next 10 years trapped in her own emotional confinement—powerless to live, yet powerless to die. When she died at the age of 82, I was in sixth grade.

Born in British-occupied eastern India, in what was then East Bengal, Grandma came from a well-to-do family. But the 1940s were troubled times. Revolt was brewing from all corners. Subhas Chandra Bose, a maverick who pledged armed resistance against the rulers, captured the imagination of the masses and Grandma joined the fight, thundering the podium against the political atrocities of the British. She donated all her jewellery and wealth in pursuit of freedom. The retaliation was quick and decisive. Her husband, a renowned gynaecologist, was stripped of his state job. In one stroke, a family of eight plunged into abject poverty. Very soon after, my grandfather died. A widow at the age of 42, with six half-fed children, Grandma decided to cross into West Bengal.

What she did next was remarkable and quite unthinkable for those times. While working and raising her children almost single-handedly, Didun turned to writing during her free time, devoting herself to writing stories, verses and songs. Schools adopted her stories and publishers loved her free-flowing rhythmic verses.[1] Didun's children became respected professionals in their various fields. She did not need to find a second companion. Books had become her retreat and refuge.

I could not fathom what happened to my Didun and perhaps the need to find the answers remained in my subconscious. Years later, well into my medical journey, I wondered at the suddenness of it all. How could a brain of such superior intellect shut down so quickly? What triggered such an agonizing collapse? Did my grandmother see it coming?

As I tried to unravel the puzzle, I realized there were many others who grappled with equally painful circumstances.

~

The first hushed hint of this disease was when Chandana's father bowed down to offer *pranams* to someone 10 years younger. Chandana, who was then a college student and now a close acquaintance of mine, found this behaviour odd, bizarre and grossly out of place, for her father was a man of impeccable

---

[1]*Brajamadhuri*, The Radiant Process, 1964.

etiquette. Nothing could go wrong with a man whom she always looked up to—a metallurgy engineer who worked in a private firm; someone who revelled in French movies and Rabindra Sangeet; a man of prime habits who would be dressed proper even at the unlikeliest hour.

When that same man walked out one day, wearing an unbuttoned shirt and a loosely fit pyjama, the alarm bells were sounded. A family riding high on the shoulders of a man, refined, successful and disciplined, stumbled on the road. Things went to the wire when he was found trying to stop a whirling ceiling fan with his bare hands. A screaming mother sought out Chandaṇa who rushed and pulled her father down seconds before a probable blood bath.

Clueless doctors poured in clueless opinions. He was in his mid-60s. The traditional dump of dementia did not fit the bill for Saswata Chatterjee. What followed next was probable psychotic behaviour, depression, schizophrenia, and so on. His expressionless stare betrayed all emotions. The sockets held a pair of eyes, captive as if, unable to smile, yet unable to tear.

An astute young doctor looked at those dead eyes and floated the concept of Alzheimer's. The city's best neurologist was summoned. He scribbled a prescription, spoke little and disappeared. Later, from his Egyptian hieroglyphs-styled handwriting, the word 'Alzheimer's' could be deciphered. Why didn't he mention the diagnosis to the family? What prevented him from discussing the possibility of Mr Chatterjee suffering from Alzheimer's? What was so dreadful about that word? Or was it that he simply did not care? We will never know the answers, for he never came back.

Helpless, a family watched the collapse of a gentleman, stripped of all emotions, activities and dignity. With no specific methods of diagnosis during the 1990s, and with no specific nursing homes meant for Alzheimer's patients, he was shifted to a city hospital in Calcutta for better care. The move turned out to be disastrous, as there was a lack of fundamental medical ethics, and not even the basics of comfort could be provided. Chandana's father returned home with a gaping bed sore.

He might have lived in a vegetable state years ahead as many others who got swallowed by this disease did. However, his suffering was short. He choked on a dinner table one dreadful evening. The food particles entered the lungs. He was rushed to the Intensive Care Unit (ICU). He never recovered from the aspiration pneumonia. He passed away eventually, a pathetic exit from a stage he had always graced with poise and elan.

~

Dr Bharati Sharma was one of those destined to be different and brilliant. An outstanding student in India, she boarded a plane to England at a time when women in medicine were few and far between. Despite her scholarly excellence, Dr Sharma had little idea that her own brain would sink into Alzheimer's, grounding a mind that prided itself on taking care of mothers and infants in distress.

A single word announced the arrival of Alzheimer's. In a letter to her husband, she started off normally, with 'My dear husband', but as the letter progressed, quite suddenly and with no heralding sign, she lost her way and stumbled to a halt after a paragraph or two, ending the letter with 'Yours affectionately, Mother'.

A disease, at a frenzied pace, reversed her identity in a matter of a few lines. There was no turning back. A doctor turned into a patient who would need to be taken care of for the next 20 years. All was lost, except tragic remembrances, like when she scrubbed her hands, surgeon style, every time she sat for dinner—painful reminders that she was once an outstanding doctor.

These examples bring out the nature of Alzheimer's: unreliable and unsure. How much of the mind it bites away and how much it chooses to spare seems to be entirely left to the discretion of its whims. No matter how we try to formalize its ferocity with guidelines and templates, a new version inevitably emerges from behind the curve.

The three examples describe the tone of this disease: at once unpredictable, complex and uneven. Inevitable questions arise. When did it surface amongst us? When was it first recognized? Or was it always with us? Can we anticipate its advent? Can we cure it? And if we can't, can we prevent it?

INTRODUCTION

THE STORY OF DR ALOIS ALZHEIMER AND AUGUSTE DETER

Dementia carries a long lineage, maybe a lineage as long as the human civilization. While today's socially sensitive thinkers protest the derogatory connotation of the word 'demented', the world fared far worse, centuries ago, when science was struggling to find its foothold. Unsurprisingly, hundreds and thousands of those whose minds faltered prematurely were termed as witches and burned alive. Goaded by superstitions, religious bigotry and false presumptions, men and women perished the moment their intellects got displaced from the norm.

Yet, dementia wasn't unknown to the stalwarts of science. From Greek mathematician Pythagoras to the Father of Modern Medicine, Hippocrates, senility and cognitive disorders were acknowledged scientifically. Much later, as medicine matured and theocracy retreated, dementia became formally recognized as a medical disorder. Through the hands of illustrious names like the French doctor Philippe Pinel and his disciple Jean-Étienne Dominique Esquirol, to German scientist Emil Kraepelin and his disciple Alois Alzheimer, dementia was expressed variously as a consequence of old age, stroke, syphilis, brain tumour and other relentlessly evolving pathologies.

The birth of Alzheimer's disease was noted through a woman named Auguste Deter. A seamstress assistant, Auguste married Karl Deter in 1873 and settled down in Frankfurt, Germany. The couple had a daughter, whom they named Thekla. Time flowed without a ripple till March 1901, when Auguste started to act odd. She abruptly accused her husband of adultery, became careless with her housework, lost her ability to cook, started to forget and misplace things, forgot how to write, dragged a bedsheet out in the open, cried her heart out during midnights and became agitated at the slightest pretext…all these in a span of a few months. At the age of 51, on 25 November, the same year, Auguste Deter entered the Frankfurt Mental Hospital under the care of Dr Alois Alzheimer's.

Her mental and emotional fluctuations continued in the hospital. While she could recognize and identify objects like pens, cigarettes and keys, she thought she ate spinach, when she actually had cauliflower and pork. She arched between offensive comments to extreme politeness, stone still silence to midnight cries. She needed to be placed in a bath filled with water to calm her agitations and had to be locked up at night to abort her wandering temptations.

Dr Alzheimer's chronicled all these activities, summarized all her aspects of memory loss and dysfunctional conditions in the minutest details and came to the conclusion of 'presenile dementia'.

Five years later, on 8 April 1906, pneumonia ended her suffering, as she succumbed to the infection at the age of 55. History will remain indebted to her husband Karl for allowing Dr Alzheimer to study his wife's brain. He was then in Munich. Soon after Auguste's death, her brain was sent from Frankfurt to Munich, along with all other medical records. On receipt, without a minute to spare, Dr Alzheimer set to conduct the biopsy of her brain.

For the first time in medical history, an Alzheimer's patient's brain was studied. Auguste's cortex was found to be thinned. All the regions of the brain, involving the ones controlling memory, language, judgement and thinking, were found to be severely impaired. Plaques and tangles were found in the nerve fibre. A dreadful disease had announced its presence.

More than a century later, with far more advanced imaging studies and far deeper understanding of science behind the disease, we are still searching for the light at the end of the tunnel.

WHY THE MEDICAL WORLD FACES ITS DARKEST HOUR IN ALZHEIMER'S DISEASE

Nowhere is the cry for answers more poignant than with Alzheimer's disease. A terrifying spectacle sinks mind after mind, unbridled and untouched by any type of resistance thrown in its way. This disease springs from an organ that is the least understood, one that robs a person of emotion and identity, transforming all humane faculties into an expressionless stare.

In Alzheimer's disease, the medical world is facing its darkest hour. Of all the diseases that continue to harass humanity, Alzheimer's holds hostage the very fulcrum of human existence: its mind. Far more surreptitious than a stroke or tumour that grows, flares or strikes with characteristic visibility and ferocity, Alzheimer's is that serpent in the grass that doesn't give a hint of its existence. Its deceptive presence evokes virtually no resistance, as it spews its venom remaining virtually unchallenged. When it finally decides to announce itself, the human brain has already turned into jelly, helpless to the serpent's sinking teeth.

Scientists and physicians have tried to defy the disease the way they always have—with imaging studies, molecular genetics and pharmaceutical industries. But we also realize that unlike other disorders that harp on certain organic traits, Alzheimer's deals with memory, the finest of our faculties. For an entity as integral, infinite and invisible as memory, a drug or a procedure is as futile and redundant as a group of ants trying to grapple with a giant pizza.

So, while stress can be managed, mood can be elevated, growth can be arrested, blood can be stalled and a clot can be busted, memory cannot be revived with a single magic pill.

The chatty familiarity of care, love and affection do little to dent the fact that when it comes to cut-and-dry disease prevention, today's practice of medicine is still scratching the surface. Unlike any other organ, the brain remains the only one that has little control over the boundless possibilities of its own existence. Moving from consciousness and awareness to motivation, intention, insight and free will, the brain and mind arc seamlessly back and forth, exchanging each other's position as cause and effect.

Like the classical Achilles heels of modern medicine, Alzheimer's disease highlights the shortcomings and incredible challenges of a branch of science that, despite its rapid advances, thrives on external discoveries while completely ignoring the treasures from its own internal resources. The understanding that this disease is much more than a rusty brain that has dwarfed due to disuse, makes one gawk at the limitless possibilities that might be leading to this tragic state of inertia. The overwhelming fact remains that unless we have a deeper understanding of how the mortal mind works beyond the configuration of the brain's anatomical landmarks, we will find it hard to tame a beast that revels in random invasions. In other words, unless we comprehend how we remember and relate, we cannot comprehend how we forget.

What makes matters more ominous is the rapidly emerging concept that Alzheimer's is neither just about loss of memory nor does it involve only the sufferer. Almost like an infectious disease, it trespasses from the patient to the caregiver. The sheer emotional trauma of caring for a loved one who is physically intact but functionally defunct is bound to wreck the emotional mind. With mounting evidence showing trauma and stress as major risk factors, caregivers themselves become potential victims of this disease. A singular disease turns into a family affair that is at once vicious and aggressive. As a result, depression, agitation, personality changes, stress and allied cognitive disorders become inevitable ingredients of a complete package for both the patient and the caregivers. For a disease of such ruthless pervading nature, it is myopic to think of a solitary or a singular approach.

To put it succinctly, this is one fiend whose taming calls out for not just neuroscientists but masters of philosophy, sociology, physics and, I dare add, spirituality.

FRIGHTFUL STATISTICS IN ALZHEIMER'S DISEASE: INDIA AND THE WORLD

Let us move to facts and figures because numbers tend not to lie. Simple statistics will tell us that we are at the threshold of an epidemic. Someone in the world develops dementia every three seconds. According to Alzheimer's Disease International, there were over 55 million people worldwide living with dementia in 2020. This number is predicted to almost double every 20 years, reaching a staggering 78 million in 2030 and 139 million in 2050.[1] Current research from the National Institute on Aging estimates that between 2010 and 2050, the number of people aged 65 and older will more than double to 88.5 million, or 20 per cent of the population. Emerging as the most populated country in the world, India faces a grim situation. Statistically, about 8.8 million Indians, living above the age of 60, have dementia.[2] By 2050, people aged 60 and above are predicted to constitute approximately 19.1 per cent of the population. These would make an excess of 14 million people with dementia by 2050.[3] This could very well be

---

[1]'Dementia Statistics', *Alzheimer's Disease International*, https://tinyurl.com/527e69c6. Accessed on 29 November 2023.

[2]Lee, Jinkook, et al., 'Prevalence of Dementia in India: National and State Estimates from a Nationwide Study', *Alzheimer's and Dementia: The Journal of the Alzheimer's Association*, Vol. 19, No. 7, July 2023, pp. 2757–3251.

[3]Ravindranath, Vijayalakshmi, and Jonas S. Sundarkumar, 'Changing Demography and the Challenge of Dementia in India', *Nature Reviews Neurology*, Vol. 17, 2021, pp. 747–58, https://tinyurl.com/4vmj8798. Accessed on 29 November 2023.

an underestimate, as there is no formal nationally estimated study in the country. We are thus facing a tsunami, completely unaware and unprepared.

WHY INDIA FACES AN UPHILL TASK IN TACKLING ALZHEIMER'S

On a deeper look at the state of Alzheimer's care in India, one can clearly see that the reality is dark and ominous. Due to lack of an inherent nationwide research infrastructure, prospective or retrospective epidemiological studies, we have little understanding of the root causes of Alzheimer's, specifically in the context of the Indian population. Information to trace vascular risk factors (like diabetes, high blood pressure and high cholesterol), gender and genetic influences on the prevalence and progression of dementia is scarce. Any clinical cure or care becomes farcical if lacking research endorsement.

While India's incredible cultural diversity is the world's envy, its demographic diversity offers a daunting task to the scientists when it comes to the field of epidemiology (the branch of medicine which deals with the incidence, distribution and possible control of diseases and other factors relating to health). Studies[4] show that major disease distributions differ widely between various states, urban and rural areas. Despite scientific progress, well-meaning governmental policies and endless sprouting of non-government organizations (NGOs), India remains a country where warmth, luxury and comfort lie side by side with cold, starvation and poverty. Alzheimer's reaps from both ends of this unhealthy spectrum—malnourishment and immunocompromise of the poor; and obesity and diabetes of the affluent. India is home to

---

[4]Basu, J., 'Research on Disparities in Primary Health Care in Rural versus Urban Areas: Select Perspectives', *International Journal of Environmental Research and Public Health*, Vol. 19, No. 12, 2010, pp. 7110.

77 million adults with diabetes[5] and forms one of the epicentres of this disease. Parallel high incidences of high blood pressure and high cholesterol make the situation even more explosive. Both public and private sectors have endeavoured genetic studies to track vulnerable genes for the disease. For a country with such disparity and diversity, these are bound to be time consuming and expensive. The utter dearth of nursing homes or trained healthcare providers sensitive to Alzheimer's patients is thus an expected but agonizing reality.

It will not be out of place to mention that Alzheimer's is not the only form of dementia that exists. Closely related forms like Lewy Body Dementia, Parkinson's Related Dementia, Frontotemporal Dementia (FTD), among many others, are increasingly recognized with overlapping pathologies and features, adding to the challenges. In India, many of these get diagnosed and dismissed as age-related dementia.[6]

BASIC MANIFESTATIONS OF ALZHEIMER'S DEMENTIA: A BIRD'S-EYE VIEW

So, what exactly constitutes Alzheimer's—an aggressive and most common type of dementia? Despite the variability and the complexity of this disorder, there are certain characteristics that stand out as fundamental and intrinsic.

As a full-blown syndrome, Alzheimer's encompasses the following:

- Slow gradual onset
- Progressive worsening

---

[5]'Diabetes in India', *World Health Organization*, https://tinyurl.com/3d7xywky. Accessed on 29 November 2023.

[6]Lee, Jinkook, et al., 'Prevalence of Dementia in India: National and State Estimates from a Nationwide Study', *Alzheimer's and Dementia: The Journal of the Alzheimer's Association*, Vol. 19, No. 7, July 2023, pp. 2757–3251.

- A decline from a previous level of functioning and performing
- Interference in the ability to function at work or in carrying out day-to-day chores
- Cognitive impairment, which impacts acquiring and remembering new information; reasoning and handling of complex tasks; language, personality and behaviour changes
- Predominant amnestic presentation (impairment in learning and recalling recently learned information)
- Predominant non-amnestic presentations, including language presentations with word-finding deficits, visual-cognitive deficits and dysexecutive presentations

HURLING DEFIANCE AGAINST DEMENTIA

Sensing a disaster, scientists, clinicians, nurses, social workers and all other healthcare providers shook hands to confront this beastly household disease. We have sharpened our skills to sense the drift of a disease far away; anticipated hushed steps of a predator; invented various ways to sharpen our memory skills; learned how best to take care of our Alzheimer's patients by creating the right ambience, the most structurally compatible rooms and nursing homes; and how to take care of our exhausted caregivers.

We have turned to music for solace and sustenance. Drug-shy scientists continue to push the boundary and happily venture into the realms of music and its eclectic effects. We delve into intriguing studies that emphasize the beneficial effects of music for our cognitive processing. We undertake the fascinating journey of Mozart's 'Sonata for Two Pianos' in D Major on cognitive aspects of the human brain (the so-called Mozart Effect) and, in the process, discover that music can become a surprising friend to the lost mind.

We have the pharmaceutical industry-approved drugs specifically for the treatment of Alzheimer's, like donepezil, galantamine, rivastigmine and, very recently, lecanemab came in. They rolled in with great expectations, carrying loads of promises while riding on various hypotheses that tinker with the brain's neurotransmitters. Each took their own turn being bestsellers, and yet how none have been able to halt Alzheimer's in its relentless, destructive march.

Thus, it became imperative to go beyond pharmaceutical industries and seek solutions from holistic avenues. We realize that in India, with all its internal and inherent demographic challenges, implementations of such holistic interventions would be easily adaptable and scalable, as they can easily circumvent literacy and economic frictions.

Among all these invigorating concepts, meditation and yoga, both steeped in centuries of experience, quickly took root. What began as spiritual practices, from the deep recluses of mountains and forests, soon promised firm pathways of human relief. As an inward journey, meditation took a completely different path to address various cognitive challenges.

But what has lifted them to the level of serious consideration is the recognition of the major risk factors behind Alzheimer's. The understanding of stress, high blood pressure, high cholesterol, obesity, diabetes and family history as strong risk factors for Alzheimer's remains a firm point of entry when it comes to grappling with the disease.

This is precisely where and why yoga and meditation emerge as helping hands—with both being observant and insightful. Modern times foster a lifestyle that spirals us out of our own existence. We seem to have lost the restrained elegance of a purposeful life. Nowhere are those helping hands needed more than now.

Much scientific evidence has begun to show that meditation can rewire brain circuits to produce calming effects, not just on the mind and brain but also on the entire body.

In many ways, German psychiatrist Hans Berger can be considered as the father of twenty-first century neuroscience. The founder of the electroencephalogram and the discoverer of various brain waves, Dr Berger opened the floodgate of a field of research that until then had drawn little attention beyond derision and ridicule. What started off as an electrocorticogram on a 17-year-old boy on 6 July 1924, became a mind-bending gateway to explore the human brain.[7]

Meditation and all forms of holistic medicine before Berger were at best a cult—an oriental ritual lacking science and sophistication. In the early days of the century, when the first faint trickle of the benefits of meditation reached the scientific society, there was nothing too cerebral to boast of in the world of technology to detect the 'sick states' of a brain. Computed Tomography (CT) scan, sophisticated version of Magnetic Resonance Imaging (MRI) or Positron Emission Tomograms (PET) were still a far cry at that time.

Unlike any other pharmaceutical drugs, the very fact that these techniques can endorse neuroplasticity (ability to form new nerves) on centres of focus and attention, and increase alpha waves (responsible for enhanced cerebral attention and poise) make them superior options for treating a disease for which the world has little answer.

The sounding board came from Dr John Denninger, director of research at the Benson-Henry Institute for Mind Body Medicine at Massachusetts General Hospital. A strong advocate of meditation and yoga for wellness, he cited the works of Dr Herbert Benson from Harvard Medical School, whose landmark research paper showed decreased oxygen consumption, increased carbon dioxide elimination and higher respiratory rate, among other parameters—

---

[7]Tudor, Mario, Lorainne Tudor and Katarina Ivana Tudor, '[Hans Berger (1873-1941)—The History of Electroencephalography]', *Croatian Academy of Medical Sciences*, Vol. 59, No. 4, 2005, pp. 307–13.

all indicators of a state of sustained calm—in those who practiced meditation.[8]

'They certainly suggest benefits,' Dr Denninger said. 'What is really needed is a "longitudinal study" comparing minds with and without the practice of meditation. That would find gold.'

Dr Benjamin R. Doolittle, Yale's program director of Combined Internal Medicine Pediatrics Residency Program, goes even further. He laments the fact that meditation, despite all that has been researched, is still an offering or option that is entertained only at the very late stage of a disorder.

For long, we have meditated for our spiritual well-being. For long, we have labelled meditation as a religious exercise. For long, we have wrapped it under the cover of endless rituals. Time has arrived to bring it under the microscope, know its intricacies, its immeasurable depth, its scientific and practical capability to prevent many an ailment.

Suddenly, an audacious question beckons: Not as a spiritual practice, certainly not as a religious ritual, can't we prescribe meditation as hardcore scientifically approved guideline to prevent Alzheimer's?

A cursory look around, spanning across national boundaries, up mountain ranges, or deep into forest recluses, will reveal similar postures, soaked in demure composure and echoless silence. These men and women live long and with complete mastery over their minds and emotions—a grand display that entices us to not only revisit their microcosm but also lure them to our medical fraternity as healers of our mind and soul.

I have ended the book, talking about the challenges related to the disease, how to take care, with a strong emphasis on the concept of prevention. In tackling Alzheimer's, prevention

---

[8]Wallace, R.K., H. Benson and A.F. Wilson, 'A Wakeful Hypometabolic Physiologic State', *The American Journal of Physiology*, Vol. 221, No. 3, 1971, pp. 795–9.

forms an essential aspect, specifically when we realize that we are still struggling with the evolving pathologies of the disease, let alone having a firm therapeutic cure. The redoubtable eye of the storm has been the emerging concept of Mild Cognitive Impairment (MCI)—a prelude to the ultimate tragic drama. It is the phase where the disease is still in its infancy, thus giving an opportunity to nip it in the bud before the fatal explosion.

To me, and many of us, the pivotal aspect of our health lies in prevention. It becomes imperative when we realize that in the hands of time, physical decay is inevitable. An attempt should be made to make our natural degeneration as graceful and painless as possible. If we prevent the risk factors from becoming a disease, we can end with minimal physical and emotional pain. Our exit does not have to be so tragic.

ONE

WAYS AND MEANS TO KEEP YOUR MEMORY STRONG

'Gratitude is the memory of the heart.'

—Jean Baptiste Massieu, French bishop

TWO MAJOR MEMORY TYPES DESTROYED BY ALZHEIMER'S

Alzheimer's inflicts functional damages on working and declarative memory. While the former is all about performance, the latter (also called explicit memory) deals with recollections.

It will not be out of place to probe deeper into these aspects, not just for better appreciation of their relevance but also to seek opportunities to rehearse and solidify their presence. Rather than getting into tedious definitions of their various ramifications, some prime examples will serve the purpose.

A person with an intact working memory will be able to follow the sequence of events, while keeping the basic story in mind. They will remember the address of a location while driving through the detailed pathways. In other words, their short-term memory can be implemented into a coordinated and coercive action.

A declarative or an explicit memory, in contrast, deals with remembering experiences, events and facts. In other words, what did you have for dinner last Tuesday? Or what is the capital of Gujarat?

Alzheimer's starts its silent voyage into our minds by impacting these two. The consequences are slow but sure, sinking into our brain, layer by layer. And when it turns its eyes from objects to human faces, all hell breaks loose. That's when relationships collapse, families break—a suffering hitherto unknown and unanticipated takes centre stage.

How do we stop this slide? More importantly, how do we anticipate a slide before it actually begins? Subconsciously, and inevitably, we circle back to the pivotal word of this book, 'prevention'. To put it succinctly, we humans must use all our mighty forces to prevent memory from melting into a useless cesspool.

In this context, it will help us to remind ourselves that Alzheimer's is an entirely different kind of a beast that is at once nonlinear and nondescript, a nonconformist that will refuse to follow the trodden path. In simple but harsh terms, it means that die hard scholars and professors can fall under its radar, just as farmers and janitors who have never read a line (let alone a book) cannot escape its wrath.

That being said, we will reach for the lowest hanging fruit, grab the single standing straw or clutch onto the last handful of sand to make sure that those two types of memories are kept as strong as possible. Simply put, we must lock and bolt our entrances, to thwart any possible invasion, today or tomorrow. Let's deal with some of them.

FIRM HANDSHAKE[1]

Handshakes have existed for centuries. Its genesis lies hidden in the haze of time. Some historians refer to it as a gesture that was meant to be weaponless and hence peaceful. Others pointed to the

[1]Loprinzi, Paul. D., et al., 'Handedness, Grip Strength, and Memory Function: Considerations by Biological Sex', *Medicina*, Vol. 55, No. 8, 2019, pp. 444, https://tinyurl.com/yrwhe3j6. Accessed on 29 November 2023.

up and down motion as further proof that no swords were curled inside one's sleeves. And there were those who called it a simple goodwill gesture. Nevertheless, handshake evidences were found in the relics with earliest depictions found in a ninth century BC relief, showing the Assyrian King Shalmaneser III pressing the flesh of his hand with a Babylonian ruler to presumably seal an alliance. Later, handshake motifs were found both in the Greek and Roman civilizations.

While regular handshakes as a customary courtesy appears to have been born from the Quakers, the subsequent Victorians willed for a gentle handshake rather than a firm and a rough press.

What an irony, that in today's world, a firm handshake has been positively associated with better memory recall performance. While the exact neurological pathway is yet to be firmly established, strong circumstantial evidences do point out to memory-enhancing effects of a firm handshake.[2]

LEARNING DIFFERENT LANGUAGES

One does not have to know Powell Janulus, Kató Lomb, Kenneth Hale or, the crown of all, Giuseppe Caspar Mezzofanti, the figures etched in history as master polyglots. A look into our own rich Indian history will unveil names like Harinath De, Swami Rambhadracharya, Ali Manikfan, Pramathanath Banerjee as hyperpolyglots, in essence, masters of many languages.

Why are we bothering ourselves with these names? Simply because, overwhelming research[3] approves learning different

[2]Jin, Ya-Li, et al., 'Association of Hand Grip Strength with Mild Cognitive Impairment in Middle-Aged and Older People in Guangzhou Biobank Cohort Study', *International Journal of Environmental Research and Public Health*, Vol. 19, No. 11, 2022, p. 6464.

[3]Schroeder, Scott R., and Viorica Marian, 'A Bilingual Advantage for Episodic Memory in Older Adults', *Journal of Cognitive Psychology*, Vol. 24, No. 5, 2012, pp. 591–601.

languages as a definitive tool for enhancing episodic memory—a type of memory that recalls recent and past events, like remembering a pleasant experience a decade back, or breakfast contents from a day before.

India, in that context, is blessed. According to the People's Linguistic Survey of India, we have the second highest number of languages and dialects (780) after Papa New Guinea (839).[4] We could have had more, but according to a survey by the Vadodora-based Bhasha Research and Publication Centre, we have lost 20 per cent of our languages in the last 50 years following the disappearance of various nomadic communities that we had harbored for centuries.[5]

Despite the losses, there is one blessing at our doorstep. Unlike most countries, India has 22 different official languages. Even a cursory attempt to imbibe the various languages will be a guaranteed boost to our memory reserves. To make matters even better, this boost is not age sensitive. One can be nine or 90. It's never too late.

GET A GOOD NIGHT'S SLEEP

> *'Innocent sleep. Sleep that soothes away all our worries. Sleep that puts each day to rest. Sleep that relieves the weary laborer and heals hurt minds. Sleep, the main course in life's feast, and the most nourishing.'*
>
> —*Macbeth*, William Shakespeare

---

[4]G. Seetharaman, 'Seven Decades after Independence, Many Small Languages in India Face Extinction Threat', *The Economic Times*, 13 August 2017, https://tinyurl.com/mrx5pwrp. Accessed on 29 November 2023.

[5]Soman, Sandhya, 'India Lost 220 Languages in Last 50 Years, Survey Finds', *The Times of India*, 9 August 2013, https://tinyurl.com/2cuj48m7. Accessed on 29 November 2023.

All of Shakespeare's quotes turn out to be not just profound and time–transcending but also objectively scientific. Sleep and its benefits are no exceptions to the rule.

Adequate sleep, in fact, helps in all three aspects of a memory, be it acquisition (getting new information), consolidation (stability of a memory formed) or recall (ability to access the newly formed memory). Scientists believe that characteristic brain waves during various sleep stages, like Rapid Eye Movement Sleep (REM) or Slow Wave Sleep (SWS), help in creating new memories.[6] Further research delved deeper to prove that both declarative memory, like remembering past events or experiences, and procedural memory, like remembering to play the piano notes or riding a horse, are strengthened after a good night's sleep.[7]

How much is a good night sleep, you might ask? Most of us say, seven to nine hours.

COLOUR CONSCIOUSNESS

This troubled phrase has a glorious exception. When it comes to memory revival, colour does matter.

Long standing and extensive literature highlights the immense benefits of specific colours when it comes to focus, attention and memory.[8] Surveys on students in preparation for educational studies showed significant memory gains when academic materials were colour coded or highlighted.[9] When compared to various methods of memorization procedures—like learning by heart, frequent revisions, supplementary video-materials, animations and colouring

---

[6]'Why Sleep Matters: Benefits of Sleep', Divison of Sleep Medicine, Harvard Medical School, https://tinyurl.com/3hup22mc. Accessed on 5 December 2023.
[7]Potkin, Katya Trudeau, and William E. Bunney, 'Jr. Sleep Improves Memory: The Effect of Sleep on Long Term Memory in Early Adolescence', *PLoS One*, Vol. 7, No. 8, 2012, https://tinyurl.com/yc8y2847. Accessed on 29 November 2023.
[8]Diachenko, Inna, et al., 'Colour Education: A Study on Methods of Influence on Memory', *Heliyon*, Vol. 8, No. 11, 2016.
[9]Ibid.

text with or without illustrations, coloring of texts produced impressive and superior recall of facts and figures. Some colours, like yellow, red and orange fared better than the others. To drive the nail home, red has been found to be the best for memory retention.[10]

From a pragmatic standpoint, we can extrapolate these findings to a broader scheme of things. How about donning colourful dresses, spreading a red tinged bed sheet on your bed or even painting your wall orange? The possibilities are limitless and fascinating.

IF YOU CAN WALK, DANCE!

This is not to take away from the tremendous benefits of walking, for some of the greatest minds in history have put their boots on the ground and walked out of passion. From Aristotle, Ludwig van Beethoven, William Wordsworth, Mary Oliver, to Henry David Thoreau, these famous men and women have worked and walked at tandem. Philosopher Søren Aabye Kierkegaard's thoughts on walking sound like that from a scientist:

> Above all, do not lose your desire to walk. Every day, I walk myself into a state of well-being and walk away from every illness. I have walked myself into my best thoughts, and I know of no thought so burdensome that one cannot walk away from it. But by sitting still, and the more one sits still, the closer one comes to feeling ill. Thus, if one just keeps on walking, everything will be all right.[11]

---

[10]Zavaruieva, Inna, Larysa Bondarenko and Olha Fedko, 'The Role of Colour Coding of Educational Materials When Studying Grammatical Categories of the Ukrainian Language by Foreign Students', *Review of Education*, Vol. 10, 2022; Castro-Alonso, J.C., et al., 'Learning Symbols from Permanent and Transient Visual Presentations: Don't Overplay the Hand', *Computers and Education*, Vol. 116, 2018, pp. 1–13.

[11]'Søren Kierkegaard Quotes', *The Cite Site*, https://tinyurl.com/2a9cb3bp. Accessed on 30 November 2023.

However, it is dance that has caught the roving eyes of science. Studied among other leisure activities as possible factors to lessen impending dementia, dance has been singled out as one of the most cogent preventive measures from an impending dementia.[12] Scientists went deeper to find out that dance increased 'neuroplasticity' (a term denoting increased nerve growth) and also boosted cross connection between both the cerebral hemispheres (either of the two hollow convoluted lateral halves of the cerebrum).[13]

As for what type of dance styles auger best for our memory, whether it is Kuchipudi, Odissi, Bharatnatyam, salsa, polka or ballad, that's for the future pundits to ponder. As for now, move your feet, swing your arms and shake your hips.

SMARTPHONES: FRIEND OR FOE?

Taking a casual look into the scientific literature, one would be flooded with anecdotes, notes, papers, thesis, table talks, seminars, conferences, name what you may, all vilifying the atrocities of a gadget called smartphone. The world is full of news about how smartphones distract the young minds, shrinks the attention span, creates a disease called Attention-Deficit/Hyperactive Disorder (ADHD), blunts one's imaginative power and eventually enslaves you to an audacious palm size object.

But we have a caveat here. These smartphones are here to stay—just as the apple that fell from the tree or the light bulb

---

[12]Marie, Damien, et al., 'Music Interventions in 132 Healthy Older Adults Enhance Cerebellar Grey Matter and Auditory Working Memory, Despite General Brain Atrophy', *Neuroimage: Reports*, Vol. 3, No. 2, 2023, https://tinyurl.com/32v44tnt. Accessed on 30 November 2023.

[13]Teixeira-Machado, Lavinia, Ricardo Mario Arida and Jair de Jesus Mari, 'Dance for Neuroplasticity: A Descriptive Systematic Review', *Neuroscience & Biobehavioral Reviews,* Vol. 96, 2019, pp. 232–40, https://tinyurl.com/ycx8byn6. Accessed on 10 December 2023.

that Edison introduced. These are objects that shorten oceans and bridges, brings stadiums to our bedrooms, calls taxis to our doorsteps, brings a mother to a son, in short, defines our modern lives. It is a unique Catch-22 situation, where Dr Jekyll and Mr Hyde reside in the same room, side by side.

Scientists from University College London and New York University forged a study to break the ice.[14] Contrary to the popular notion that smartphones give rise to 'digital dementia' (a popular term alluding to a lazy brain overdependent on a plethora of information fed to the brain), their conjoined study showed that individuals hooked to smartphones showed far better attention and memory than those without digital dependence. This outstandingly daredevil verdict comes from the scientific understanding that the brain actually frees up its memory space once it knows that some routine information is stored in the gadget. Instead of going dull, it does the very opposite. With remarkable alacrity, the brain rewires to selectively preserve other events and experiences, taking full advantage of a gadget that takes care of the other mundane chores. To give a succinct example, when we are selecting the best available restaurants downtown, the brain will use the stored options in the smartphone to make the subtle decision as to which one is ideal in terms of accessibility, location, traffic conditions, cuisine choices, price range and internal ambience.

Where do we stand now? To my mind, we are facing a healthy problem. A problem where the solution is in our hands. If intelligently handled, we can use smartphones as an external aid to free up our memory cells, and use them to remember events and experiences that we *want* to remember.

---

[14]Dupont, D. Q. Zhu, and S.J. Gilbert, 'Value-Based Routing of Delayed Intentions into Brain-Based Versus External Memory Stores', *Journal of Experimental Psychology: General*, Vol. 152, No. 1, 2023, pp. 175–187, https://tinyurl.com/y47msswj. Accessed on 30 November 2023.

WHAT'S ON YOUR PLATE?

As per the World Health Organization (WHO) guidelines, balanced nutrition holds the key to physical and mental well-being.[15] For a lean meat-eating race though, I do not have good news. Almost every clinical study[16] points to memory-declining characteristic of meat, be it beef, pork, lamb or duck. But, what should an ideal memory-boosting plate look like? Daggers are drawn at the idea of 'Western diet', which consists of high consumption of refined, processed foods, saturated fat, trans-fat and sugars, along with a low intake of fruits and vegetables. Make no mistake. Western diet is not restricted to Western countries. The eastern part of the world, including India, devours as much of the Western diet as their neighbours across the ocean.

Backed by enough scientific evidence, the Mediterranean diet has been the darling of the healthy. Comprising high quotient of fruits, vegetables, whole grains, fibre, nuts, legumes and olive oil, the diet goes low on consumption of sugars, saturated fat, red and processed meats, and industrialized foods.[17] In addition, decreased incidences of Alzheimer's have been observed with increased fish consumption.[18] From a host of vitamins and minerals, vitamin D

---

[15]FAO, IFAD, UNICEF, WFP, WHO, 'The State of Food Security and Nutrition in the World 2020: *Food and Agriculture Organization of the United Nations*', *Food and Agriculture Organization of the United Nations*, 2020, https://tinyurl.com/48x67uex. Accessed on 30 November 2023.

[16]Zhang, H. et al., 'Meat Consumption, Cognitive Function and Disorders: A Systematic Review with Narrative Synthesis and Meta-Analysis', Nutrients, Vol. 12, No. 5, 2024, p. 1528; Grant, W.B., 'Using Multicountry Ecological and Observational Studies to Determine Dietary Risk Factors for Alzheimer's Disease', *Journal of the American College of Nutrition*, Vol. 35, No. 5, 2016, pp. 476–89.

[17]K.V., Sandhu, et al., 'Feeding the Microbiota-Gut-Brain Axis: Diet, Microbiome, and Neuropsychiatry', *Translational Research: The Journal of Laboratory and Clinical Medicine*, Vol. 179, 2017, pp. 223–44.

[18]Morris, Martha Clare, et al., 'Consumption of Fish and N-3 Fatty Acids and Risk of Incident Alzheimer Disease', *Archives of Neurology*, Vol. 60, No. 7, 2003, pp. 940–6.

has hogged the limelight with firm incidences of mental impairment in cases that reported severe deficiency of the vitamin.[19]

What about drinks? While red wine in measured amount has been proposed as brain protective, both coffee and green tea seem to have the backing of the researchers.[20]

To recap, what are the best dietary options to preserve our brain? As of now, we will settle for a Mediterranean diet, not more than two cups of daily coffee or green tea, measured wine, vitamin D fortifications, if found deficient, seafood consumption and restricted lean meat or processed food consumption.

If you are justifiably obsessed with the right diet, a visit to the nutritionist's office is a must.

CHESS, CROSSWORD PUZZLES AND SOCIAL GATHERINGS

Though chess, puzzles and social gatherings have been known for being traditional brain activities, none of them have been proved to override an impending dementia. My father-in-law, an expert chess player, spent the last few years of his life with ever-deepening dementia. My grandmother, a scholar, an author and a social activist who thundered the political podium, got devoured by Alzheimer's in her 80s. But who knows what would have happened if chess was not played, if a book was not written? It is quite possible the disease would have swallowed them years earlier.

---

[19]Jia, Jingya, et al., 'Effects of Vitamin D Supplementation on Cognitive Function and Blood Aβ-Related Biomarkers in Older Adults with Alzheimer's Disease: A Randomised, Double-Blind, Placebo-Controlled Trial', *Journal of Neurology, Neurosurgery and Psychiatry,* Vol. 90, No. 12, 2019, pp. 1347–52.

[20]Prasanth, Mani Iyer, et al., 'A Review of the Role of Green Tea *(Camellia Sinensis)* in Antiphotoaging, Stress Resistance, Neuroprotection, and Autophagy', *Nutrients*, Vol. 11, No. 2, 2019, p. 474, https://tinyurl.com/y557uer7. Accessed on 30 November 2023.

Thus, academic exercise of any nature must continue throughout our lives. If you cannot read a book, then talk to someone. If you do not have a loved one to talk to, write a love letter to yourself. If you have a set of eyes, look deep. If you have nothing to look at…wink!

History repeats itself. What was consumption in the nineteenth century is Alzheimer's of the twenty-first. When Victorian poet John Keats coughed out blood, he famously yet poignantly had remarked, 'That is blood from my mouth…I know the colour of that blood—it is arterial blood…that drop of blood is my death-warrant—I must die.'[21]

In Alzheimer's, we face suffering, insurmountable and relentless, sometimes weeks, sometimes months, sometimes years before death. We must do all that we have in our power to prevent a fatal invasion.

---

[21]'Wentworth Place, Hampstead', *Mapping Keat's Progress: A Critical Chronology*, https://tinyurl.com/3he6nkmx. Accessed on 30 November 2023.

TWO

HOW TO TAKE CARE OF ALZHEIMER'S PATIENT

'I am seeking, I am not lost. I am forgetful, I am not gone.'

—Joanne Koenig Coste, author, lecturer and outspoken advocate for Alzheimer's disease

In my 25 years of providing patient care to those suffering from Alzheimer's, I have taken care of many helpless souls in nursing homes. I have seen them at terminal stages in ICUs. I have made home visits. I have held their hands till they would fall asleep. I have spent a day in the sun till a patient's expressionless lips curled into a smile. And almost always, I felt they knew who I was, through their stone wall façade.

Humanity is an immense gift, resplendent and ceaseless. No disease or disorder can totally silence its presence. Words can be halted, memories can be muffled, motions can be restricted, but emotions cannot be completely annihilated. They may not fall in place, they may not have an outlet, they may be miles away from the surface, but they are there, even if faint and elusive, like the last stream on Mother Earth with a barely audible trickle. There lies the strength of our hope, the solid brick of our treatment.

As a disease, Alzheimer's is a punch that knocks out the basic lighthouse of our presence—recognition. Failure to recognize the road back home, failure to identify your favourite coffee, failure to fathom those eyes that forever nurtured you…and finally, failure to recognize oneself. This final point of destruction is what makes this disease inexorable and inexhaustible. This very 'unawareness' of one's own incapacity, one's own forgetfulness, one's own intractable well of suffering call for an insurmountable duet between the patient and the doctor.

So vast is the untraversed territory and so deep is the unfamiliarity that when it comes to Alzheimer's, all of us are doctors. All of us, from the direct caregiver to each and every member of a family, to the social worker of an institution, to the passerby who rescues the stranded patient, to the window that lets in the sunlight, to the landscape with its persuasive warmth, all become the doctor in need.

So, how do you take care of your mother, father, brother or sister suffering from Alzheimer's? Before that, let me rehearse and get into certain details of the gamut of aberrant emotions the patient might be going through.

PROVOKING FACTORS BEHIND BEHAVIOURAL SYMPTOMS OF AN ALZHEIMER'S PATIENT

The two extreme actions that engulf an Alzheimer's patient are agitation and apathy. I prefer to call them reactions, especially when it comes to agitation. Invariably, they are reactions to stress, and that could come from anywhere. Truth be told, the stress threshold gets invariably lowered as the disease progresses. What makes it more challenging is that when dementia deepens, coping mechanisms weaken. The most subtle shade of stress, like someone talking loudly, a radio or TV blaring meaninglessly, a telephone shriek or a noisy room, can provoke an agitated reaction.

Bathing is often a challenge. It is a daily chore that has the potential to evoke a stressful reaction. A refreshing diurnal ritual for the intact brain can turn into a frightful experience for those suffering with dementia. Even a change in water temperature can provoke agitation. Conveying discomfort through words gets replaced by an agitated gesture, or in some cases even a violent action.

How does apathy set in? This, too, is a reaction. A bottled-up emotion sets in when repeated agitation turns useless and redundant. The frequent episodes of 'wandering away' are also a reactive need to walk away from a stressful situation, be it in their family home or a residential facility.

Clutter or any visual chaos form another set of stress-provoking situations. It teases the brain that is already submerged in internal chaos. Same goes for enclosures. Any narrow space leads to an overwhelming sense of claustrophobia that is guaranteed to incite unrest. Similarly, locking the room or applying physical restraints are bound to negatively affect mood and desire for social interaction.

Why is it important to identify these factors? It is simply necessary because understanding these trigger factors will help us create the apt social and environmental ambience needed to reduce or eliminate the aberrant reactions. Such ambiences assume supreme importance when we realize that it will reduce unnecessary use of antipsychotic and other psychotropic medications that are useless and detrimental. Evidences clearly show that indiscriminate use of drugs (rampantly used in India and many other countries) increases the risk of stroke, heart attacks and overall mortality.

In fact, formal guidelines state that antipsychotic drugs can be prescribed in situations of extreme violence wherein the patient or the caregiver is in a state of danger, but only after medical, physical, functional, psychological, emotional, psychiatric, social and environmental causes have been identified and addressed.

SIMPLE MEASURES, PROFOUND EFFECTS

Before getting into the specificities, it is imperative to remind ourselves that merely removing the discomforting situation or source is not akin to giving a comfortable ambience—precisely because each patient of Alzheimer's is unique in their struggle, complexity and suffering. Thus, a cookie-cutter, one-size-fits-all, perfunctory method is inadequate and downright disrespectful. In Alzheimer's, an individualistic approach must be adopted.

Broadly speaking, medical and environmental measures need to be taken into consideration. They are exclusive, yet entwined, mutually leaning on each other.

One watchword applicable to anyone suffering from any disorder is calmness. In the context of Alzheimer's alone, it becomes mainstream. A calm hand, a calm voice, calm utterances, a calm room can form the very basic infrastructure on which medical or environmental management can be launched.

MEDICAL MANAGEMENT: SENSORY PRACTICES

Scented Oils

With growing evidence showing positive link between smell and memory, the scent of oils extracted from seed, bark, stems, roots and flowers have been found to have an overall phlegmatic effect.[1] Once exposed to the soothing aroma, positive memories (happy memories) are kindled, invariably leading to an elevated mood. As its route of administration is indirect, the acceptance rate has been predictably high. A number of studies[2] have highlighted the benefits of aromatherapy in decreasing aggression and agitation in individuals with dementia. Whether administered using room diffusion, sachets, a patch or as a skin cream, the calming effects have been remarkable nonetheless. While large-scale efficacy

[1]Press-Sandler, Olga, et al., 'Aromatherapy for the Treatment of Patients with Behavioral and Psychological Symptoms of Dementia: A Descriptive Analysis of RCTs', *Journal of Alternative and Complementary Medicine*, Vol. 22, No. 6, 2016, pp. 422–28.

[2]'Aromatherapy, Massage and Dementia', Alzheimer's Society, https://tinyurl.com/ycykk59h. Accessed on 5 December 2023.

trials are on the way, some studies[3] have already shown a direct beneficial effect on the brain.

Massage

This is an ancient practice, time-tested and well-researched. However, I will be a bit cautious here, as not all Alzheimer's patients are or will be receptive to massages. This is essentially a tactile approach that is at once individualistic and subjective. But if receptive, its benefits are strong, various and long-lasting. As a non-verbal means of communication, it helps diffuse a stark social isolation that engulfs an Alzheimer's patient. A sense of company, comfort and care follow along with evidence-based results of decreased agitation, aggression, stress, anxiety, depression and disruptive vocalizations.[4]

In a residential facility, massage emerges as a powerful tool of connection and relationship when a patient sunk in dementia turns more vulnerable in an unknown territory. A gentle massage not only serves as a harmless, gentle, unobtrusive introduction but also as a firm reassurance that helplessness need not be felt alone.

What are the most rewarding areas of massage? Again, it becomes subjective and patient-specific. In general, however, massaging the back, shoulders, neck, hands or lower legs and feet have shown maximum benefits. The diverse techniques, be it slow or large strokes, rubbing, kneading or even acupressure allow one to cater to a patient's comfort zone.

Just that touch: A forgotten treatment

Palm on a palm, hand on a shoulder, sublime feel of a caress—all reach infinitely deep beneath the skin. Once a hand is held or a

---

[3]Ibid.

[4]Behrman, Sophie, Leonidas Chouliaras and Klaus P. Ebmeier, 'Considering the Senses in the Diagnosis and Management of Dementia, *Maturitas*, Vol. 77, No. 4, 2014, pp. 305–10.

shoulder is touched, countless emotions surge forward from the sudden rush of an awakened heart.[5]

While in conversation once with Dr Constante Gil, the programme director during my residency and a mentor who has shaped my medical journey, the topic drifted towards the importance and absolute necessity of touch in Alzheimer's treatment. He mentioned his daughter's experiment on the sublime effects of touch on newborn babies. Dr Karla Gil, a paediatrician in Florida, researched the beneficial effects of massage on preterm babies. It included soft, subtle and gentle touch. The babies would roll over in unspoken ecstasy. The results were amazing. These preterm babies gained the optimal weight required for discharge much earlier than those receiving 'sham massage' (a lighter-pressure caress that does not blanch the skin, as opposed to the massage that provides just enough pressure to blanch the skin where it is touched).

It is of little wonder that a connection as profound as touching captures the interest of scientists. The temptation comes from other areas, too. Here is a form of treatment that costs nothing, is easily reproducible, creates no untoward reactions and—perhaps most important—carries none of the dangers of a drug intake, namely adverse effects, resistance and tolerance.

But what are we aiming to achieve by 'touching' an Alzheimer's patient? Here, we should remind ourselves again that these hapless victims suffer from more than loss of memory. As part of what we call the behavioural and psychological symptoms of dementia (BPSD), a patient deals with a gamut of emotions, such as an expanding range of agitation, aberrant motor behaviours (including wandering away and irascibility), hallucinations, anxiety, depression, apathy, delusions and sleep alterations. As strong components of the

[5]Gleeson, M., and F. Timmins, 'The Use of Touch to Enhance Nursing Care of Older Person in Long-Term Mental Health Care Facilities', *Journal of Psychiatric and Mental Health Nursing*, Vol. 11, No. 5, 2004, pp. 541–45.

disease spectrum, any or all of these become important prognostic factors in a patient's impaired functional activities, which become even more pronounced when the sufferer faces abject isolation in nursing home and allied facilities.

Several studies have demonstrated that almost all Alzheimer's patients have experienced at least one episode of these allied BPSD at some point during their illness. The Cache County Study on Memory Health and Aging[6], a collaborative research endeavour comprising scientists from Utah State University, Duke University Medical Center and Johns Hopkins, examined the genetic and environmental factors associated with the risk of Alzheimer's and other forms of dementia.

One of their studies conclusively showed that 97 per cent of a cohort of 408 patients with dementia experienced at least one behavioural or psychological symptom. As expected, the five-year prevalence was highest with depression (77 per cent), followed by apathy (71 per cent) and anxiety (62 per cent).[7] Various ranges of behavioural aberrations tended to club together, like wandering with sleep problems or irritability with persecutory delusions.

Touch works to ameliorate these behavioural symptoms. As expected, we are not looking at generic, gentle random touches as modes of management. In fact, various supervised and guided forms of these non-pharmacological interventions have been developed. Some of these fall under emotion-oriented therapies; others are a part of the sensory stimulation interventions, including massage or touch therapy, while many belong to functional analysis-based interventions and exercise therapy.

---

[6]Tschanz, J.T., et al., 'The Cache County Study on Memory in Aging: Factors Affecting Risk of Alzheimer's Disease and Its Progression after Onset', *International Review of Psychiatry*, Vol. 25, No. 6, 2013, pp. 673–85, https://tinyurl.com/mst3exwa. Accessed on 30 November 2023.

[7]Tschanz, Joann T., 'A Population Study of Alzheimer's Disease: Findings from the Cache County Study on Memory, Health, and Aging', *Journal of Care Management,* Vol. 6, No. 2, 2005, pp. 107–14.

Almost three decades ago, scientists M. Eaton, I.L. Mitchell-Bonair and E. Friedmann E. evaluated the effect of gentle touch on 42 institutionalized patients diagnosed with what was then called 'chronic organic brain syndrome'.[8] An innovative and fascinating method of measure was adopted in the study: nutritional intake.

In this trial, patients were randomly assigned to experimental and control groups. Nutritional intake was evaluated for three consecutive weeks. During weeks one and three, all patients were encouraged to eat. In the treatment (second) week, the experimental group members received gentle touches along with verbal encouragement. The results were fascinating. Food intake was significantly greater in the experimental group compared to the control group during the other two weeks. The researchers had every scientific right to proclaim that, as a simple intervention, 'tactile stimulation' can be implemented for these patients as a viable adjunct to verbal encouragement.

Ruth Remington, from the University of Massachusetts, studied the effects of calming music and hand massage on patients with dementia.[9] The goal was to demonstrate whether these non-pharmacological interventions had any effect in decreasing agitation, as is often found in these cohorts of patients. Four sections were created among 68 patients who suffered from various types of dementia, including Alzheimer's, multi-infarct or senile dementia. They were exposed to calming music and massage, either separately or simultaneously, and no intervention. Each of these lasted 10 minutes and was given once to each patient.

The treatment effect on 'agitation level' was evaluated by using the standard, modified version of the Cohen-Mansfield

---

[8]Eaton, M., I.L. Mitchell-Bonair and E. Friedmann E., 'The Effect of Touch on Nutritional Intake of Chronic Organic Brain Syndrome Patients', *Journal of Gerontology*, Vol. 41, No. 5, 1986, pp. 611-6.

[9]Remington, Ruth, 'Calming Music and Hand Massage with Agitated Elderly', *Nursing Research,* Vol. 51, No. 5, 2002, pp. 317–23.

Agitation Inventory (CMAI), administered by trained research assistants who, whenever possible, were blinded during treatment allocation.[10]

The results clearly showed that each of the experimental interventions reduced agitation, compared to the group that received no intervention. The benefit of reduced agitation was sustained up to one hour following the interventions.

I remain leery of scientific tools when it comes to measuring the success of these subjective avenues of hope. More research should follow. Some will meet the criteria for validity, while others will fail as scientific evidence—just as meditation, music and other holistic approaches did.

Until then, if holding their hand extracts the faintest smile from your beloved sunk in dementia, keep holding on for a few more minutes. I am reminded of a patient of mine at a nursing home in North Carolina. She was then 92 years old and had been suffering from Alzheimer's for the last 10 years. She would simply sit on her bed side chair and stare meaninglessly into nothing. Every time I visited her, I would draw another chair, sit across her and hold her hands. One afternoon, a miracle happened. She squeezed my hand and smiled graciously.

PSYCHOSOCIAL PRACTICES

Validation Therapy, Power and Potential of the Right Spoken Word

This, to me, is the pillar of our management: respecting and acknowledging the present state of being without any deception or domination; realizing that behind a demented mind, there might be an intact heart; realizing that in between clouded thoughts,

[10]Cohen-Mansfield Agitation Inventory is a 29-item questionnaire designed to measure the types and frequencies of agitated behaviours exhibited by elderly nursing home residents.

emotions are alive. They may lack the connectivity or the seamless transition from one faculty to another, but they are present. They may be held back or subjugated, but again, they are there.[11]

The word 'patient' sometimes robs the 'human' aspect of the being. In our desire to master the organ at fault, we dismiss the 'person'. We label far too often. We label the smile of a person with dementia as meaningless. How do we know it is meaningless? Why can't it be a sign of self-dignity, so as not to be dismissed as 'demented', or a valiant act of self-defence or self-preservation? To put it unabashedly, why can't the 'meaninglessness' of that smile be a reflection of our own ineptitude and inability to decipher rather than being the sufferer's shortcoming?

In other words, that unhealthy domination of intactness over presumed incapability of a disease must come to an end. Only then can two human beings converse and connect, not always as a dialogue between a provider and a patient.

In Alzheimer's, words, tone and attitude play a pivotal role. Words that are non-threatening, understanding, spoken with empathy, gently and in an unhurried pace hold value.

In a nursing facility, or even at home, a gentle knock before entering is probably the first wordless show of respect that can set the ball rolling. Expectations must be rolled back, for one is addressing a human being far more vulnerable, unsure and overtly sensitive. How about greeting that person by their name? How about rephrasing the person's jumbled words as a show of understanding, or responding in general terms when meanings are unclear?

Always greet an Alzheimer's patient with their name. Include them in decision-making even if their responses are inadequate (like asking what food they enjoy). Collaborate and work as a

---

[11]Livingston, G., et al., 'Systematic Review of Psychological Approaches to the Management of Neuropsychiatric Symptoms of Dementia', *The American Journal of Psychiatry*, Vol. 162, No. 11, 2005, pp. 1996–2021.

team for uncomfortable activities, in a way that those become comfortable for the person (like giving a bath or helping them get dressed). Encourage and promote self-expression or independent activities. Let them share a joke, even if childish, or let them gift a present to a dear one. Recognize and acknowledge any accomplishment, howsoever small and trivial, by clapping, smiling or singing. Give them space to relax (like listening to music or walking). Give them company when they are in distress, not by rectifying but rather through rationalizing the grievance or cause of agitation. Always endorse creativity (like spontaneous dancing, singing or gardening).

Never treat a patient like a child, disregard a word or an expression that fails your understanding. Do not start conversing to a third person, dropping your conversation with the patient midway. Never take advantage of their forgetfulness and manipulate an answer. Always avoid rushing with your truckload of information or choices.

REMINISCENCE THERAPY

Who doesn't like remembering fond memories? Who doesn't like flipping through an old, tainted photo album while sitting by the midnight lamp? Who doesn't like recalling that exquisite piece of music that had once taken the young, undaunted mind by storm?

Nothing should change when it comes to an Alzheimer's patient. Mounting evidence shows increased well-being, pleasure and cognitive stimulation from recalling past events. The basic understanding is that older memories are more enduring than recent ones.[12]

[12]Cabrera, E., et al., 'Non-pharmacological Interventions as a Best Practice Strategy in People with Dementia Living in Nursing Homes: A Systematic Review', *European Geriatric Medicine*, Vol. 6, No. 2, 2015, pp. 134–50.

Reminiscence therapy can be implemented in various ways and, as mentioned before, it must be person-specific. Accordingly, it can be an individual recollection or a part of a group session. Similarly, the mode can be either free recall (through conversation), based on specific stimuli (through photograph or music) or a life-review method (creating a chronological life sketch book). One word of caution here. Never ask a patient to identify an object or recognize a face. To someone whose memory and sense of identification is lost, these questions are hurtful and counterproductive. At the worst, their dignity is hurt. On the contrary, reinforce their memory by identifying those things by yourself.

POWER OF THE PRESENT: MEANINGFUL TAILORED ACTIVITIES

Let us take a fresh look at our beloved ones drowned in Alzheimer's. For them, their past lies in a rubble of disjointed thoughts and emotions. Suddenly devoid of recognitions and relationships, a future becomes non-existent for them. While we try to garner all our resources to seek a semblance of order for them, a priceless box of treasure goes unnoticed. The sufferer's very moment of existence.

Indeed, the power and profundity of the present is frequently overlooked by humans, who are forever reminiscing the past and rushing for the future. For an individual with Alzheimer's, a preoccupied present often holds the key to an enhanced quality of life. Science is of the firm belief that while agitation or verbal disequilibrium (like speaking out or screaming) are outcomes of social and medical mismanagement, apathy or nonchalance stem from lack of 'using' the present. And the only way of using the present is to engage in meaningful activities.

What exactly do we mean by meaningful activities? They can range from complex tasks involving many steps (making salad, simple woodwork, designing a table) to one-to-two steps task (sorting beads, playing ball with grandchildren) and sensory-based tasks (video viewing, listening to music).

And how do these activities help? Activities replace the void and a vacuous obedience that can only deepen dementia. They enhance role identity, and promote self-expression and positive feelings. A grip over one's identity takes place.

PET THERAPY

How many times have we seen the heart-melting picture of a golden retriever or a labrador of colossal size snuggling close to an infant in sound, undisturbed sleep? How many times have we watched them locked in a world of ecstasy, each feeding the other with boundless, immersive joy?

Emotional power of an unspoken, uneven, unrelated love forges a bond that is inexplicable yet fulfilling. For decades, pet therapy has been the guardian angel for the terminally ill, people with physical and emotional difficulties and the lonely and elderly. A strange, sixth sense prevails among domesticated dogs and cats, and it draws them towards humans less perfect and yet more complete.[13]

That being said, this therapy, like some others, needs to be patient-specific. We must keep in mind allergic reactions, hygiene concerns and agitation issues for those patients who have had negative experiences with animals in the past.

---

[13]Bernabei, V., et al., 'Animal-Assisted Interventions for Elderly Patients Affected by Dementia or Psychiatric Disorders: A Review', *Journal of Psychiatric Research*, Vol. 47, No. 6, 2013, pp. 762–73.

STRUCTURED PROTOCOLS, CHALLENGES AND REMEDIES[14]

Mouth Care and Bathing

Why am I highlighting these two activities among all others? A closer look into the intricacies of these activities will shed light on the reason. Think about mouth care, of which regular brushing forms the fulcrum. One is looking at an intimate affair for which the patient with Alzheimer's is now dependent on a stranger. To the mind in the thick of dementia, this is an intrusive undertaking based on unknown hands trying to access their face and teeth. A negative reaction becomes almost justified, be it refusal to open the mouth, clamping on the toothbrush, or plain and simple hitting out. It is a confrontation that is inevitable. It does not surprise us that in most nursing home facilities, oral and dental care takes a backseat. The obvious outcome is that a person with dementia will likely develop oral hygiene issues, mouth ulcers and dental infections.

Keep in mind that brushing their teeth is another activity that demands person-specific approach. To begin with, a designated time and caregiver is important. Unlike the general population, an Alzheimer's patient may not want brushing to be the first activity after waking. Thus, we need to patiently find out a time that is conducive to the person's mood. Remember, as mentioned before, brushing is an intrusive job, which is why trust is an important ingredient in this activity. Let us now get into the details.

While gentle, unhurried and slow-motion techniques are obvious, some more specific approaches are preferred. Approaching

---

[14]Zimmerman, Sheryl, et al., 'Systematic Review: Effective Characteristics of Nursing Homes and Other Residential Long-Term Care Settings for People with Dementia', *Journal of the American Geriatrics Society*, Vol. 61, No. 8, 2012, pp. 1399–1409.

from the front, asking for permission, explaining the procedure while performing it, keeping a smiling and friendly face, giving constant encouragement comprise the basics.

What happens when the patient concerned refuses mouth care or simply refuses to open their mouth? That's when patience takes centre stage. That's when we need to try to understand the reason behind the refusal. Is it pain? Is it wrong timing? Or, is it just unaccountable, unfounded fear? A deeper insight will tell us that all these are modifiable factors, and hence correctable. Make a note of the perfect timing. Be patient and cooperative while trying to mitigate fear of pain or fear of the unknown. Demonstrate the technique on your own teeth. Distract them with TV, singing, small talk or keeping the hands preoccupied with some other objects. You can also defer the task, and come back when the patient is feeling better and is conducive to your efforts.

When it comes to bathing, reactions have been far more dramatic with evidences of screaming and hitting out. It is not difficult to comprehend how and why water becomes a fearful object for the mind that has lost rationality. Hydrophobia is as reasonable for a mind that has lost the ability to recognize things as it is for the child who does not know how to swim. Without proper understanding and training, bathing thus becomes a distressing activity for both the patient and the caregiver.[15]

Let us turn to the right modes of bathing. With many past examples pointing to increased agitation associated with cold water bath and direct shower spray, recent interventions conducive to Alzheimer's patients have adopted a more person-specific and empathetic approach. Quite like mouth care, the preliminary care

[15]Gozalo, Pedro, et al., 'Effect of the Bathing without a Battle Training Intervention on Bathing-Associated Physical and Verbal Outcomes in Nursing Home Residents with Dementia: A Randomized Crossover Diffusion Study', *Journal of the American Geriatrics Society*, Vol. 62, No. 5, 2014, pp. 797—804, https://tinyurl.com/ms3rbswb. Accessed on 11 December 2023.

must entail gentle caress, calm approach with explanations and pleasant distractions, like small talk, singing, soft music and use of scents. To get into further details, multiple evidences have shown that the sequential use of covering the body with bath blankets, gently running warm water over the body, then replacing bath blankets with towels, followed by gentle massages have yielded calmer reactions.

Dressing

Two words will encompass the concept of ideal attire when it comes to dressing your loved one, now sunk in forgetfulness: compatibility and comfort. Imagine the emotional challenge for a mother or a grandmother, deep in dementia who once took delight and pride in the gaudy dresses she wore, the jewellery she flaunted, the stilettoes that graced the floor. We will have to be objective here. What will matter in the end is how she feels presently, what will make her happy presently and what will not make her agitated and give her emotional trauma. We, the caregivers, will have to keep in mind that our reactions are less important than their forgetfulness. We will act exactly the way they will warrant us to act. In other words, if comfort is what is warranted, then dresses need to be that much comfortable and compatible.

My experience has shown that loose fitting clothes cause minimal anxiety. A garment that can be put on and taken off easily or will cause minimum restrictions is ideal. I have written about compatible colours, like light blue or light green. However, these rules are not set in stone. Let them be compatible to their likings. Let us not experiment with our choices. Familiarity is comforting in forgetfulness. The same coloured clothing, the same soothing textured materials, the same comfortable socks and slip on shoes or sandals are likely to be more acceptable. In that context, buttons and zippers may be unnecessary hindrances. How about a one-pull track suit?

Bottom line must remain the same: it's about their choice and comfort.

Feeding

Quite like bathing, feeding can be challenging. This challenge can only be circumvented by compassion, creativity and loads of patience. To the Indian palate used to curries, spices and curds, we must simplify and adjust. Let me now give a step-by-step guide about the feeding process.

Let us be subjective at every step. Just because a grandfather loved watching soccer while eating, once upon a time, does not mean that the same ritual has to be enacted at a time when he has lost his normal bearing on life. In fact, a blaring television or a radio can be a big distraction. A soothing instrumental music might help. Lighting needs to be bright without being glaring. A round table is a far better option than a rectangular table with sharp edges. Firm, comfortable chairs will help. Table mats with loud colours will provoke anxiety. On the contrary, light colours will soothe the tensed nerves. However, a colour contrast with the main dish plate will be required. It will not help matters to have a white plate on a white mat. Invariably, the mat will be used as a plate.

What about the act of feeding? Depending on the stages of dementia, the process has to be slow and personal. As mentioned before, like bathing, feeding has been known to cause anxiety and agitation. The feeding process thus has to be an art that will first and foremost cater to a patient's comfort. Forks, of course, must be religiously avoided. Soup spoons are usually to the liking for most patients struggling with fancy cutleries. But if fingers are preferred, then be it!

What type of food? Again, his or her preference takes precedence. A word of caution here. In Alzheimer's, especially in the advanced stage, difficulty in swallowing can occur. Thus, spicy and hot foods, large chunks of any food or a lavish spoonful of curry is inadvisable. For the vegetable lovers, chopped soft pieces of cucumber, carrots, beetroot and cabbage are easily digestible. Fish (strictly without bones) and poached egg preparations are good non-vegetarian options. Chicken soup (as opposed to chicken pieces that can notoriously get stuck in the throat) also has a very high acceptance rate.

During any feeding time, be it breakfast, lunch or dinner, company is a prerequisite. Eating alone becomes an arduous task. Smooth, soft talk, light jokes, a bit of smile and laughter, and eating together, will invariably make the process wholesome and pleasurable. Be it bathing, dressing or feeding, these activities warrant more of art than science. Compassionate, emotional and creative hands would be far more compatible than just regimented and objective steps.

VIRTUAL REALITY

How Home Came to Andrea

Andrea kept the nurses on their toes. Admitted with Alzheimer's, she showed frequent displays of emotional outbursts, ranging from agitation to incessant crying spells. It was getting impossible for her brother, five years her senior, to handle Andrea. She was obviously not compliant with her medications. Although she had recovered most of her motor strength from a stroke three years earlier, her original self had not recovered. Since then, she had also undergone a hemicraniotomy to remove a brain tumour.

Andrea threw a fit at everything offered to her, and, in between, displayed a smile that seemed more of a neurological aberration than a symbol of happiness.

Psychiatrists did their part, but Andrea revelled in her negativity, refusing to take any medication, any vitamins or any nutritional supplements.

'Would you like to have your food?' asked one of the nurses, pleading with Andrea.

'No!'

'You did not take your blood pressure medications, Andrea. You need to take them.'

'Hell, NO!'

I made more emergency visits than routine ones. Andrea would be given haloperidol by the psychiatrist to curb her hostility but to no avail. She would fall asleep, but the moment haloperidol's effect would wane, she would revert to her trademark 'No!' echoing through the corridors.

Once, while entering her room, the nurse whispered to me.

'During surgery, I am sure the surgeon must have removed her "yes" centre. Good lord, she says "no" to everything.'

Andrea looked at me with frosty eyes. From her unkempt appearance, it was evident she was under a perennial storm. Her gown was half-open, her hair dishevelled and her parched lips twisted sideways. She looked every bit like a hostage in restraints. I smiled back. She did not return the pleasantry. I completely bypassed the usual formalities. I found it fruitless to inquire how she was doing, and instead asked softly, 'Sweetheart, would you like to go home?'

She whispered back instantly. 'Yes!'

'How on earth am I supposed to tackle her, now that you promised her home?' the nurse said in an exasperated tone. 'You are not discharging her, right?'

'How about bringing home to her?' I said, before explaining the destructive effects of an adjustment disorder, how it can totally derail someone's personality and worsen any ailments.

We soon called up Brent, Andrea's brother. I explained her condition and requested some details of the room she had been occupying before her transfer to our facility. Brent texted me a photo of her room. An exact replica was impossible in a nursing home. Instead, we procured all the pictures that were in her room at home—pictures of her grandchildren; of her only son in his graduation gown; of herself when she was young, arm in arm with her husband, both smiling away on a ship deck; and many others.

We moved Andrea to a different room. It was brightly lit with sunlight filtering in. The window on the eastern side of her room commanded a majestic view of a valley, immersed in green. All her photographs were kept on the side table by her head.

As she entered her new room for the first time, she looked intently at the photographs and suddenly turned back.

'Where is Debbie?' she asked, referring to her granddaughter.

Before I could muster a response, the nurse responded, her emotions pouring out, 'She will be coming, Andrea. They all will be coming.'

The example cited here is all about introducing familiarity to a mind trapped in an alien ambience. This is called Simulated Presence Therapy (SPT), and has been extended further to be called 'simulated family presence therapy'. It is based on the observation that nursing home residents who are more frequently visited by family members exhibit less agitation and greater life satisfaction. It first came to our attention in 1995.[16] Patricia Woods and Jane Ashley, both registered nurses from Massachusetts, conducted research with 27 nursing home residents suffering from dementia. They all listened to an audiotape prepared by their caregivers. The results showed a substantial reduction in behavioural problems and less manifestation of verbal aggression. The choking feeling of social isolation was lessened and there was a refreshing increase in positive behaviours, including better verbalization, smiling and singing.

The seeds of virtual reality are sown in this very concept.

As the name suggests, walking a mind through a virtual realm intricately close to reality is what virtual reality therapy entails.

---

[16]Woods, P., and J. Ashley, 'Simulated Presence Therapy: Using Selected Memories to Manage Problem Behaviors in Alzheimer's Disease Patients', *Geriatric Nursing*, Vol. 16, No. 1, 1995, pp. 914.

It is now becoming a tool for healthcare professionals to address depression and dementia.

The opportunity and capability to live virtually through an experience, oscillating from a sublime scene to a thrilling motion, are at once rejuvenating and refreshing. Mood elevation is almost a guaranteed denouement. As John Keats wrote in his poem, 'Endymion', 'A thing of beauty is a joy forever', likewise, beauty can be infused in the brain, pretty much like feeding a baby. To the depressed mind or those incapable of extracting beauty from a masterpiece, be it a framed piece of art or a cadenza, virtual reality can become the ideal guide to joy—pristine and free of complication.

Soniya Kim, a physician in the San Francisco Bay area, made her depressed patients and those suffering from dementia wear headsets. The results were as mood-elevating as any evidence-based approach. She mentioned how a six-foot, two-inch tall male patient, 'hunched over and constantly anxious', reluctant to enter into any conversation, solo or in a group, started singing and flapping his fingers when he 'experienced' the trajectory of a bird in the virtual reality programme. Noticing his visible transformation, his wife burst into tears.[17]

Other than evoking joy and happiness, can virtual reality be used to revive lost memory? Can Andrea's sudden recollection be reproduced in greater density through an even more vivid display of her past life? In short, can Andrea's past life be duplicated and brought back to her? This is an incredible stretch of the imagination, which is gaining foothold in modern science.

Nowhere is this as hotly pursued as in Australia. Like other countries, Australia has been hit hard by Alzheimer's, with more than 409,273 Australians currently inflicted with dementia, a figure that is expected to rise to 400,000 in less than five years.

---

[17]Platoni, Kara, 'Virtual Reality Aimed At The Elderly Finds New Fans', *NPR*, 29 June 2016, https://tinyurl.com/yb4vnhu5. Accessed on 30 November 2023.

With no breakthrough on the horizon, experts fear that the numbers may spiral as high as 771,913 by 2050.[18]

Virtual reality is not an entirely novel avenue of treatment in the field of healthcare. It is being increasingly used in robotic surgery and medical personnel training as diagnostic tools, among various other uses. The breakthrough lies in its clinical application in psychiatry. Its rewarding effects concerning emotional emanation are being entertained in various countries.

I will end this section with an incident, both emotional and thought-provoking. I was chatting with lawyer Jonathan Gray in his Manhattan office one afternoon, when he related to me this poignant moment with his 85-year-old mother suffering from advanced Alzheimer's. Jonathan was flipping through a magazine when his mother happened to look into the side mirror and apparently seeing his son's image, had shouted out, 'Jon!'

Startled and choked with emotions, Jonathan jumped to his mother's side, for it had been years since his mother had called his name, let alone recognize him.

'Mom, you know me?' Jonathan somehow whispered.

Yet, by the time, her face turned from the mirror to see her son, she had lost all sense of recognition again.

'I still hold on to that moment, Dr Sen, I still hold on to that moment.'

'It's momentary eternity, Jon,' I had replied.

What unknown nerve pathways made a mother recognize her son through an image but not in reality? I don't have an answer, but I do know that in the hands of time, momentary happenings invariably turn into gracious, scientific truths.

---

[18]'Dementia in Australia', *Australian Institute of Health and Welfare*, 21 September 2023, https://tinyurl.com/yhh3ywj4. Accessed on 30 November 2023.

ENGINEERING AND DESIGN MANAGEMENT CONDUCIVE TO AN ALZHEIMER'S PATIENT

The supreme importance of a holistic approach, coupled with traditional prescriptions, when it comes to a consummate process to slow down the onset of Alzheimer's disease becomes a necessity. To that end, not just non-pharmacological medical management but also compatible environmental and structural involvement becomes imperative. To be more precise, when it comes to Alzheimer's, patient-sensitive corridors, dining rooms, backyards, lightings, bath tubs, all possess the potential to offer care.

It is important to get into the details of the infrastructure of a house or a nursing home facility.[19] In the broader scheme of things, an I-pattern structure is preferred instead of 'L' or 'H' or square-shaped units. Residents with moderate and severe dementia fare much better and actually find an I-pattern structure more compatible to navigate when journeying to a kitchen, bedroom or toilet. Interestingly, despite various colour-coded residential floors, residents found little benefit from them, and instead relied on specific furniture or large floor numbers painted on the walls.

Small units lodging a few residents together, built and designed to reflect a home-pattern, provided more emotional cushion than large residential facilities. Thus, wall décor, coffee tables, paintings, photographs of not just loved ones but also of oneself in younger days, all reflective of what once was intimate and pleasurable, become indispensable mood elevators.

Visibility and space are further design tools that positively affect dementia patients. Not just for safety purpose and generalized mood elevation, space offers more opportunities and

[19]Chaudhury, H., et al. 'The Influence of the Physical Environment on Residents with Dementia in Long-Term Care Settings: A Review of the Empirical Literature', *The Gerontologist*, Vol. 58, No. 5, 2018.

better ambience for residents to engage in social interactions.

Dining Hall

Mealtimes are great meeting points, a confluence of various minds, thoughts and emotions. An ideal dining hall should thus reflect an ambience of togetherness and relaxation, so as not to make meeting nutritional demands a challenging task.

A structure that is cosy without being crampy fosters bondage among patients rather than sprawling spaces that easily cause distractions. Like everywhere else, a home-like décor with flowers, calendars, wall paintings of landscapes auger well for the psyche. Additional research shows beneficial effects of bright lighting and visual contrast (like using distinct colour contrast) between table mats and plates on lessening agitation and enhancing food intake and functional independence. In fact, using high contrast tableware (like red, blue and other bright coloured plates, cups and stainless-steel cutlery) produced significant intake in food and fluid intake among individuals with severe dementia rather than low contrast colours (like white and grey).

Bathing Area

Designing a compatible bathing area is of tremendous importance primarily because of the sensitive nature of diurnal routine. This is one crossroad where agitation, physical altercation, despair, dignity and respect fall in one place. Yet, simple, structural and personal changes can do wonders for both patient and caregiver.

As I had mentioned previously, shower spray, running water and abrupt, noisy splashes can be extremely detrimental to a patient's psyche. A bathroom should have a window and enough lighting. Bath tubs need to be engineered in such a way that it allows entrance from both the sides or from the end. Water temperature must be to the liking of the patient and not the caregiver.

As for toileting, commodes need to have rails on both sides, to not only prevent falls but also to enable and encourage patients to use their arms and wrists.

In general, bathrooms should be located at a visible distance from the bedroom, easily accessible with no turns and bends in between. I always advise caregivers not to rush with diapers. To me, that's cheating a patient of their ability to perform the basic necessities, howsoever restricted. Rather, make the task, as seamless and comfortable as possible.

I have strongly hinted at the acknowledgement and appreciation needed to recognize the permanence of human emotions, no matter what the disease or disorder is. Self-dignity falls in the list. Presence of multiple caregivers and unwarranted onlookers rob the patient of self-dignity. There are clear evidences that one of the prime cause of agitation and violence from patients of dementia stem from the helpless realization that they are being watched by strangers.

These are vulnerable people. Inadequacy has forced them to surrender. This is exactly the area where maximum reverence, regards and deference need to be bestowed.

Outdoor Area

Trees, plants and flowers have always been our steadfast, silent friends. They offer shadows, they give us colours and attract birds and butterflies. A garden is a prime requirement for any infrastructure. Social interactions, outdoor activities (like walking and mild exercises), uncluttering of the mind should ideally be done in a garden.

At home, bring the garden in—bring in the pots, grow the flowers, water the plants, be it on a verandah or on the windowsill. Let nature decide what is good for the mind.

DEMENTIA-FRIENDLY GUIDED MUSEUM TOURS?

With Alzheimer's, such is the gory battle, the relentless feud, the unending rain of blows, that any light demands to be viewed as a ray of hope, any breath begs to be called a sign of life. Hopes of such audacious nature emerge from the paintings of Norwegian artist Edvard Munch. How about a tour to the museums that lodge his masterpieces? Anecdotal as it may sound, dementia-friendly guided museum tours have successfully softened the suffering of patients.

Somehow, the vulnerable mind seems to connect with landscape paintings, the pageantry of sea and sky, profound but equally vulnerable. Somehow, the penetrating colours assuage the void left by lost memories, the deft strokes throb with significance in the receding mind. Somehow, the sea sweep enfolds the patient, pleasing both the eye and the mind. And in the process, a patient turns into a viewer, just like all of us, but with a different pair of eyes and ears.

I remain deeply optimistic when it comes to the power of paintings. I remember the positive impact they had on my patients. Their lips quivered, eyes sparkled, faces lit up in a see-saw of wavering resolute, trying to connect with a world, unknown but accessible.

~

THREE

WHO TAKES CARE OF THE CAREGIVER?

'Being deeply loved by someone gives you strength, while loving someone deeply gives you courage.'

—Lao Tzu, Chinese philosopher

I will begin with the father–daughter relationship I had highlighted earlier—the poignant story of Mr Saswata Chatterjee and his daughter Chandana. How a brilliant father, who was looked up to by everyone in his family, became an Alzheimer's patient, how a pampered daughter gradually turned into a caregiver and how a string of tragic events unfolded. It was a tale of reverse mentoring and indomitable courage.

CHANDANA AND HER FATHER

How do you react to a father who now fails to recognize you—a father who once was a constant sunshine over your shoulder, a father with whom you had shared endless hours watching movies, reading books, singing songs, or just sitting side by side in comfortable silence. How do you justify forgetfulness when it comes to a man who had all along guarded you like a hawk, pouncing on every tiny obstacle in your way? And worse, how do you interact? Despair? Anger? Sympathy? Exasperation? Or just veiled numbness? For Chandana, it was all of them at the same time—oscillations of a mind caught in a tempest.

One of Chandana's standout memories was her wedding night. Dressed as a bride in a resplendent red Benarasi sari, she sneaked into her father's room to change his diapers. By that time, Alzheimer's had sunk its teeth deep into Mr Chatterjee as he sat utterly oblivious of his own daughter's wedding. The much-cherished marriage rituals could never be performed by him. His brother had to step in.

Yet, strange are the ways of Alzheimer's. The following day, as the bride prepared to leave her parental house amid a wail of tears, the father broke free from his guarded enclosure, charged down the stairs and watched the final departure of his daughter in silence. No tears, no emotions. A stare that made little sense, yet somewhere, somehow, some part of the surviving brain searched for a daughter. Even for a functionless mind, the sense of anguish seemed intact. How ironic!

Many years later, Chandana's voice cracked as she narrated these agonizing moments to me.

For Chandana, the seeds of her ordeal were planted much before her wedding night. Sunk in the quicksand of ignorance and bigotry, society shied away from a family that lodged an 'insane person'. Marriage proposals had stuttered. Potential bridegrooms had hesitated to tie the knot with a brilliant woman who was also the daughter of a father 'gone mentally wrong'.

Like the tropical rain, emotional trauma can be incessant—a voracious, ever-growing appetite that gnaws the soul year by year. Relentlessly. Trauma never left Chandana, even when she bulldozed her way through life's various vicissitudes, pursued her career single-handedly and settled down in Alabama, oceans away from her seat of crisis.

WARNING SIGNS OF UNDERCOVER STRESS

So, how can one anticipate the stealthy steps of a predator? How can a caregiver sense the onrushing storm from the silence that precedes the inevitable? To be less dramatic, how would a caregiver know the stress-out signs?

Interestingly, much before the emotional breakdown, it's the body that gives out the signals. Heavy, laborious breathing, both subconscious and inexplicable, comes early. Frequently, the sensation deepens into an air hunger that wraps the lungs. Very soon, it turns into feeling out of breath at the slightest provocation. A sensation of the throat being clamped follows closely. A compensatory process of conscious swallowing makes matters worse and only increases the subjective fear of a throat closure.

Palpitation is another tell-tale sign of an impending stress—a racing heart even when you are not exerting yourself or merely thinking about a mild challenge.

Likewise, tension is a significant misery—not tension of the mind but tension of the muscles. Although, the two follow one another like cat and mouse. Tension and stiffness of the muscles of one's neck, face, shoulders and legs come next. There is a feeling of heaviness—a certain restriction in one's mobility despite no apparent cause. There is a desire to lie down as if fatigued and exhausted from a truckload of work and burden.

The transition from tension in the muscles to pain in the organs becomes inevitable. Pain in the jaw, neck, shoulders, arms—almost like a cardiac event—is a common and frightful experience typically associated with stress charging on its way. Individuals have also complained of belly pain when buckling under stress.

HOW DOES A CAREGIVER TAKE CARE OF THEMSELF

Coping Strategies[1]

Even before I get into the nitty-gritty of self-care and self-defence, it is important to differentiate between generalized anxiety and

---

[1]'Alzheimer's Caregiving: Caring for Yourself', *National Institute of Aging*, http://tinyurl.com/3at2rbud. Accessed on 12 December 2023.

caregiver's stress. These are two completely unrelated entities. While any other stress will have a strong point of entry, be it related to one's profession, financial burden, domestic or societal disputes or loss of a close one, a caregiver's trauma is totally different from the rest. It is an inherent, slow, irreversible, irreconcilable seepage of a state of mind—almost a mud-like stagnation whose source is static and relentless. While professions can be changed, finances can be improved and disputes can be settled, the trauma that comes with taking care of a loved one who has stopped recognizing anything cannot be escaped at any cost.

Thus, the usual recourse advised for stressed-out individuals—like taking a walk, watching a movie, patting your pet or making yourself a cup of green tea—are not enough for a caregiver's never-ending trauma. The remedy of a trauma that stems from the mind thus should come from the inside. A caregiver will have to trace back the same path that led them downhill.

So, what are the inescapable negative questions and thoughts that a caregiver might encounter? 'What's the use when there is no hope? How long can this thankless job continue? If only my family had escaped the disease? What's the rest of the society thinking about us? What if I get into depression? What if I come down with the same disease?'

Together, we will strive to reverse this stagnant mindset. Just as being alone is not being lonely, similarly not having a future is not akin to not having any hope. This very hard, challenging relationship does not have to be a continuation of a relationship spent in the past. This can be viewed as a new relationship where one is falling a few steps behind. There needs to be the realization of the profound fact that neither has the identity of the individuals changed nor has the love and sense of proximity between them. What has suffered is one's ability to express the intimate emotion. But deep down, it is intact.

In this regard, I am reminded of a colleague whose husband urinated in a sink instead of the toilet. Her initial exasperation was instantly replaced by her thought that at the end of the day, her husband tried to go in a 'bathroom' and not somewhere else. 'He tried. He tried,' she kept on saying, emphasizing the fact that in most situations, an attempt is as much a show of love as a complete execution.

I will appeal to all caregivers, caring for their loved ones, to go deep and feel the very care and tenderness that once had planted the bond. You may ask, what can emerge from this understanding of a bondage, unseen yet unshakable? Simply put, it is regard for love's boundless possibilities, a sense of fulfilment, a transition from self-pity to self-pride. And this is the very juncture from where renewed strength will surface—strength to challenge the instant self-grieving thoughts, strength to replace them with a mindset that is profound and assertive, strength to respect a relationship that you were always proud of.

When a Managing Partner Becomes a Caregiver

A perfect example from the above-mentioned redrawn mindset comes from Sandeep da. A senior acquaintance of mine for many years, Sandeep Roy held a coveted title under PricewaterhouseCoopers. His wife, Sneha, taught English literature to school students. They were an active, vibrant couple that enjoyed driving out to the 'cooler and calmer' outskirts of Bengal, attending classical music concerts and dining at the continental section of the Calcutta Club to escape the 'jungle of the cosmopolitan'. All these seemed seamless and smooth till Alzheimer's chose to invade Sneha without any rhyme or reason.

What started as few incidents of forgetfulness and disorientation, quickly escalated to a lifestyle-challenging event, when she had to give up driving, going to the bank, cooking, multitasking and eventually even crossing the street by herself. An upright, strong, society-conscious woman became a child in less than half a year. I saw the change in Sneha. She gradually found herself in self-confinement. She hardly spoke and would only reply in syllables. She would give a smile that could have come either from unawareness and disregard of her new disease or from the valiant efforts of a woman who was once fiercely independent. I also saw the change in Sandeep da. From despair and cluelessness to protracted silence, he went through all the phases in the initial stages. He, too, confined himself. This was a couple thrown apart by a new disease, both trying to find their way, step by step, in unchartered territories.

That's when Sandeep da broke the shackles of silence and decided to reach out. He saw no point in keeping things to himself. He talked to his friends, brought it up with his family members. He even informed his peers and the senior management of his company. We openly talked about the various options, choices and challenges that lay ahead; the available drugs in the market; their potential and futility. I advised him to go for counseling.

The way Sandeep da modified his way of life is commendable. Sneha and Saneep da are ageless lovers who are discovering news ways to love each other. As of now, the couple still goes for long walks. They still drive around. They still listen to classical music.

One night, I bumped into them at the continental section of the Calcutta Club. They were laughing and enjoying themselves. They looked engrossed in each other's company. Sandeep da was feeding Sneha. He was feeding his wife, who just needed a hand to guide her through these difficult times.

Reaching Out Strategies

Being a caregiver for someone with Alzheimer's should never be a lonely venture. Certain endeavours, howsoever noble, profound and intimate, need sharing and support. We should remind ourselves that when it comes to dementia, we are looking at a relationship where the word 'support' is essentially one-sided. Such is the nature of this disorder that even if desired and wished, the sufferer will not be able to 'support' the other. Technically, this is tangible in any terminal situation, but in dementia, the process starts from its very nascence. By the very definition of the situation, the relationship is one of a caregiver and a sufferer.

Thus, avenues of relaxation, breakout sessions and exercise are not luxuries to be indulged in but absolute necessities for emotional survival and sustenance. Of these, reaching out to support groups forms the main mode of help. Support groups include people in similar situations, professionals who are counselors, or simply friends.

Why do we need to connect with people in similar situations? The reasons are manifold. It is important to connect to others, so that you are able to share your experiences and exchange knowledge. Psychologically, advice is a great way to revisit and mend one's own identity as a sad recipient of ill-fate.

It is also important to periodically seek guidance from health counselors; to open up on challenging issues; get advice on how to address difficult situations; and how to handle yourself in the moments you feel burnt-out. Reaching out to friends, just for the sake of having a good time, is equally priceless. A session of pure, unadulterated laughter is as therapeutic as any medicine prescribed when it comes to a tired mind. On the other end of the spectrum, if required, agony or anguish of any nature also need to be released. Suffering must not be internalized. It only adds toxicity to our organs and systems. To simplify matters, bottled emotions must be unbottled to avert both emotional and physical meltdown.

Alternate Strategies[2]

Following close on the heels of the 'reaching out' strategy is the 'alternate strategy' where be it in a private home or in a nursing facility, multiple caregivers alternate in their duties. The concept

---

[2]Whitlatch, Carol J., and Silvia Orsulic-Jeras, 'Meeting the Informational, Educational, and Psychosocial Support Needs of Persons Living With Dementia and Their Family Caregivers', *The Gerontologist*, Vol. 58, No. 1, 2018, pp. S58–S73.

of caregiver shift in a professional set up is thus warranted when it comes to management of Alzheimer's. The situation turns tricky in a home when there is nobody but the elderly spouse of the Alzheimer's patient to act as the caregiver. In such situations, we need to revert to the 'reaching out' strategy, to involve all family members and discuss options of multiple caregivers within the family. Truth be told, children and grandchildren exude a very high level of acceptability from patients of dementia.[3]

I have always wondered at the dichotomy of our mindset when a child, equally vulnerable and discrete, draws so much of spontaneous togetherness as compared to the aged and those suffering from dementia, who are tossed aside to a corner bed. Both smile out of habit, both act out at the slightest challenge, both wear diapers. A shrewd society understands the power of future, the necessity of an investment and the potential of growth. The senior citizen, grounded with age and a chronic debilitating disease, will fail in all those compartments.

Even in the United States (US), research funding on Alzheimer's is peanuts compared to that of other major diseases, like cancer, cardiac attacks and stroke.[4] As a disease of the elderly, Alzheimer's garners little interest. Both intrigue and pragmatism went missing till modern times, when we suddenly realized that we are living longer.

This circles back to where I started: that when it comes to taking care of an Alzheimer's patient, all of us must be caregivers, all of us must be counselors, all of us must be doctors. A disease of such ruthless pervading nature can only be tamed by an army of caregivers.

---

[3]Alzheimer's Association, 'Alzheimer's Disease Facts and Figures', *Alzheimer's & Dementia: The Journal of Alzheimer's Association*, Vol. 12, No. 14, 2016, pp. 459–509.

[4]'Why Don't We Have a Cure for Alzheimer's?', *Alzheimer Society*, 16 July 2021, https://tinyurl.com/3f9drfkc. Accessed on 18 December 2023.

Holistic Strategies

As dealt in detail in subsequent chapters, holistic strategies embrace all modes of relaxation as is applicable for those with dementia. Quite like the patients they care for, caregivers too can benefit tremendously from meditation, music, art, physical exercise and aroma therapy.[5]

In *The Diaries of Emilio Renzi: Formative Years*, Latin American author Ricardo Piglia defined life as a combination of imposed obligations and personal moments.[6] Nowhere is this definition more applicable than in the lives of the caregivers, especially when they are caring for loved ones suffering from disorders like Alzheimer's where there is an inescapable element of a 'slow slipping away'. Personal moments thus emerge as priceless, powerful avenues of rejuvenations, a retreat, a refuge that can and must be felt and internalized to the best and fullest of one's capability.

BIDISHA AND HER PERSONAL MOMENTS

Bidisha's example comes to my mind when talking of caregivers. Growing up, idolizing her mother for all that she represented and reflected, her childhood was an uninterrupted sequence of joyful events. She had none to be envious of, her own adolescence being so replete with memories of a healthy upbringing. Her mother exuded power, personality and a starry vehemence for all that life offered her. She possessed a golden voice, sang Rabindra Sangeet fluently, displayed an eclectic taste in cooking and interior designing, and, in between, carried herself with a temperament and disposition becoming of a leader in every possible way.

---

[5]Douglas, Simon, I. James and C. Ballard, 'Non-Pharmacological Interventions in Dementia', *Advances in Psychiatric Treatment*, Vol. 10, No. 3, 2004, pp. 171–77.
[6]Piglia, Ricardo, *The Diaries of Emilio Renzi: Formative Years*, Restless Books, 2017.

When Alzheimer's did arrive, the despair and finality was unpretentious. Initial days for Bidisha were devastating, horrible and seemed irremediable. She was plunged into a new relationship with her mother. A woman who taught her about life, books and music, had turned into a stranger. The shoulder that she leaned on every second of her life was now a functionless organ. Dusted and embittered, Bidisha's self-esteem started to crack.

It was at this very juncture that Bidisha remembered one glorious gift that she had received from her mother—her ability to sing. This was one treasure that could water her drought, one treasure that could connect her to her mother, one treasure that could be indulged in and savoured.

Before she could realize, Bidisha was singing with her mother, composing songs in her private moments and singing professionally on stage.

~

FOUR

MUSIC: MIND'S MOST TRUSTED MEDICINE

'The past which is not recoverable in any other way is embedded, as if in amber, in the music, and people can regain a sense of identity...'

—Oliver Sacks, British neurologist

GLORIA SANCHEZ AND A CHRISTIAN GOSPEL

December nights are cold in New Jersey. More than a decade back, I was pursuing my residency at Raritan Bay Medical Center. As a senior resident, I was in charge of all ICU admissions. Hospital nights are a different world, ruled by silent, hushed corridors. Groans, moans and even laboured breathing emerge from the darkness. The day-long overhead pages, such as 'Code Blue', 'Code Sepsis' and 'Code Stroke', somehow dwindle in frequency. When they do occur, they scream out of a vacuum with no space for discussion. Time is tackled by the hour. Treatment is swift, objective and decisive. Patient care becomes personal. Nurses and doctors bond fiercely.

I got a page one night to see Gloria Sanchez in ICU Bed No. 5. I did not know her personally. The nurse reported that she had been having laboured breathing since the evening. Suffering from full-blown AIDS, Gloria was riddled with multiple, opportunistic infections. In those days, AIDS medications were just beginning to take shape. People still succumbed to the wrath of this disease. Not wanting to involve my two junior residents assigned for the night, I went upstairs to the ICU by myself.

Gloria was in a semi-coma. A quick look and I thought I had found the cause. Gloria's breathing problem did not stem from any respiratory issues but from a growing ascites (a fluid-filled belly, usually, but not always, secondary to a liver dysfunction). Liver failure was probably the reason behind her state.

Nonetheless, I had little option but to relieve the ascites. I instructed my ICU nurse to prepare the kit for paracentesis, the procedure to remove fluid from the abdomen. We had little chance to obtain Gloria's written permission, as her state of mind was beyond any decision-making capability. Besides, I considered it an emergency procedure.

As I suited up, I kept my cell phone on a corner shelf attached to Gloria's room. I marked the right flank of her abdomen as my point of entry. Gloria had her V-mask in place, her eyes were closed and her breathing was heavy. She flinched a little but remained unresponsive when a nurse, in a reasonably raised voice, informed her about our procedure. I was about to insert the trocar when, to my horror, I heard my phone ring. In the ongoing rush, I had not remembered to switch it off. I watched it helplessly as it rang, and was about to ask my nurse to shut it off when something that I had barely anticipated happened.

It was the night of 24 December2004, and I had set my cell phone ringer to the timeless song, 'Joy to the World'.

Midway through the tune, I noticed movement from the corner of my left eye. Gloria's eyelashes fluttered. Her eyes opened just about halfway.

'Is it Christmas, Doc?' she whispered.

'Yes, Gloria, it is,' I said. 'Merry Christmas, Gloria.'

'Merry Christmas, Doc.'

The phone stopped ringing. The music died. Gloria Sanchez went back to her unresponsive state.

THE ENIGMA OF MUSICAL PRESENCE IN OUR BRAIN

One of the most fascinating case reports in medical science came in 1997 from the Department of Psychiatry and Behavioral Sciences of the Okhaloma State University Center for Health Sciences.[1] Dr William W. Beatty and his colleagues described a patient who played the trombone and had been diagnosed with Alzheimer's about three years prior to his death from cardiac arrest. During his stay in a nursing home, the man had gradually slipped into a state of complete dependency, needing assistance in all activities of daily living. Worse, he could no longer assemble his trombone by himself. But amid all the carnage of his life, his musical skills were sustained. In what could be termed an aesthetic triumph, the man could play notes, and in some glorious moments, even brief tunes, if his trombone was assembled, placed into his hands and raised to his lips.

When he eventually died, his formalin-fixed brain was sent for microscopic examination. The brain had Alzheimer's written all over it. Very severe neuronal loss was evident in the hippocampal formation and other allied areas, along with a large number of neurofibrillary tangles and amyloid deposits.

Our trombone player goes down in history as the first reported case of Alzheimer's whose musical dexterities remained untouched, despite all other faculties shutting off in subservient obedience. Should we be surprised? Maybe not. After all, isn't music the most cardinal form of expression? Wasn't melody present millions of years before we let out the first grunt and uttered our first syllable?

---

[1]Beatty, W.W., 'Preserved Cognitive Skills in Dementia of the Alzheimer Type', *Archives of Neurology*, Vol. 51, No. 10, 1994, pp. 1040–6.

However, experts choose to explain the eternal lines of Keats, 'Heard melodies are sweet, but those unheard are sweeter.' We know for a fact that music traverses all objective expressions. Words can be formed, speeches delivered and languages mastered, yet music remains free from all such dominions, being subjective and deeply integral.

The concept of using music as a source of healing is timeless. Literature shows its evidence from Biblical days. Aristotle described music as a force that purified emotions. Hippocrates, the father of modern medicine, is said to have played music to treat his patients with mental disabilities. Thirteenth-century Arab hospitals had music rooms. In fact, music existed much before its documentation in the writings of Aristotle and Plato. Music therapy has flowed from Mesopotamia, India, Egypt, Israel and Greece, through the Middle Ages, the Renaissance, the Baroque, and into modern times.

Yet, in an age and time when belief prevailed over proof, these remained attractive propositions but with no formal backing.

OM: A SOUND THAT TRAVERSES BEYOND

Of all these, the usage of the word *'Om'* (pronounced AUM) from the ancient Indian civilization seems to have transcended antiquity and was given serious consideration as a therapy for generalized well-being.

Om does not have an exact translation. It carries an acoustic attribute that is not circumscribed by any particular organ and reportedly beckons a certain pervasive calmness. Intriguing results came from the scientists of Sipna College of Engineering and Technology in India[2], who digitized the analogue waveforms

---

[2]Gurjar, Ajay, Siddharth A. Ladhake and Ajay Purushottam Thakare, 'Analysis Of Acoustic of "OM" Chant to Study It's Effect on Nervous System', *International Journal of Computer Science and Network Security*, Vol. 9, No. 1, 2009.

of OM chanting to determine the average pitch and frequency modulation of the recorded versions.

Although rustic and lacking specific methods and materials, the experiment showed that persistent chanting of the word caused a decrease in the height of the waveforms.

Do these reflect a stabilizing effect on the brain under turmoil? A concurrent EEG (electroencephalogram), simultaneously looking into the prevalence of specific brain waves during the recording to correlate the decrease in signal amplitude, would probably be the next logical step. There are multiple avenues to probe more deeply and fully, but the study does open the gate.

Call it incidental or coincidental, but the tremendous emotional and physical benefits experienced by World War I and World War II veterans from music played by both professional and amateur musicians became an eye-opener for the medical fraternity. While Willem van de Wall pioneered the use of music therapy in state-funded facilities and authored the first music therapy text, *Music in Institutions,* E. Thayer Gaston, known as the 'father of music therapy', formally institutionalized music as a formal course of medical management.

THE MOZART EFFECT

One of the most visible, 'talk-of-the-town' musical contributions came from the famed Mozart effect.[3] Mozart's 'Sonata for Two Pianos in D major K. 448' was written in strict sonata-allegro form, with three movements. Composed in the gallant style, it featured interlocking melodies and simultaneous cadences. Intriguingly, this was one of his few compositions ever written for two pianos.

The Mozart effect started with French researcher, Alfred Tomatis who, as documented in his 1991 book *Pourquoi Mozart?*

---

[3]Jenkins, J.S., 'The Mozart Effect', *Journal of the Royal Society of Medicine*, Vol. 94, No. 4, 2001, pp. 170–2.

(*Why Mozart?*), flooded the ears of his selected patients with Mozart to presumably 'retrain' that organ at different frequencies, and eventually promote healing and development of the brain. Two years later, scientists F.H. Rauscher, G.L. Shaw and K.N. Ky, found temporary enhancement of spatial reasoning in those who listened to the Sonata, as opposed to those who underwent verbal relaxations or were not exposed to any sound at all.[4]

This set creative hearts on fire.

Lines of reasoning were effortlessly crossed, with books and articles pouring in, citing Mozart as the cure for stress, depression and anxiety—and even more fascinating—as the source of higher IQs.

An overzealous Zell Miller, erstwhile governor of Georgia, announced in January 1998 that his proposed state budget would include a whopping $105,000 annually to provide every child born in Georgia with a tape or CD of classical music.[5]

All these efforts continued till counter meta-analysis from countless scientists started to show that the Mozart effect is, in all likelihood, an artefact of arousal and heightened mood. Legislative bodies paid more attention to the credibility of the claims, with one German report concluding, 'Passively listening to Mozart—or indeed any other music you enjoy—does not make you smarter. But more studies should be done to find out whether music lessons could raise your child's IQ in the long-term.'[6]

Quite like the magic of Mozart himself, interest in these indirect effects prevailed to influence public life. As reported by *The Guardian*, a German sewage treatment plant plays Mozart to break down the waste faster, with the belief that vibrations of

---

[4]Ibid.

[5]Sack, Kevin, 'Georgia's Governor Seeks Musical Start for Babies', *The New York Times*, 15 January 1998, https://tinyurl.com/2kh9bjvu. Accessed on 5 December 2023.

[6]Abbott, Alison, 'Mozart Doesn't Make You Clever', *Nature*, 13 April 2007, http://tinyurl.com/3zmzu2rr. Accessed on 13 December 2023.

his music can just about penetrate everything—including water, sewage and cells.[7]

'The creative challenge seems to be in capturing the Mozart effect. Going by the verdict of the *Journal of the Royal Society of Medicine*, Greek composer Yanni, with his composition "Acroyali/ Standing in Motion", has done just that…with the same tempo, the same harmonic consonance, and the same predictability.'[8]

In a delightful twist, citing the same Mozart effect, researchers have proposed this classical composition as a possible cure for epileptic patents. As per the British Epilepsy Organization, listening to the piano sonata improved spatial-temporal reasoning skills and also brought down the number of seizures in people with epilepsy.[9] Research on South Carolina epileptic children found music to have a strong therapeutic effect on epilepsy.[10]

MUSIC'S JOURNEY INSIDE OUR BRAIN: FOR RESEARCH LOVERS

If you are happy just to hear the glorious success stories of music, then you can skip this section. But if you are a research buff, you will love the eclectic journey of music. Read on.

I can flood your ears with a hundred more anecdotal events underscoring the triumph of music over a disturbed mind, but it's entry into mainstream medical management can only come from firm experimental evidence. Let us study some of them to better validate our claims.

---

[7]Connolly, Kate, 'Sewage plant Plays Mozart to Stimulate Microbes', *The Guardian*, 2 June 2010, https://tinyurl.com/mryuwu4m. Accessed on 1 December 2023.

[8]Sen, Shuvendu, 'Mozart Effect and the Untapped Treasures of Indian Classical Music', *nj.com,* 28 May 2013, https://tinyurl.com/4y9tnn2k. Accessed on 1 December 2023.

[9]Ibid.

[10]Quon, R.J., et al., 'Musical Components Important for the Mozart K448 Effect in Epilepsy', *Scientific Reports*, 2021, https://tinyurl.com/2p9uw48w. Accessed on 5 December 2023.

Some of the most comprehensive research on the power of music has come from David Aldridge, Chair for Qualitative Research in Medicine, Institute for Music Therapy, University Witten Herdecke in Germany. Aldridge highlighted various anecdotal events to demonstrate that whereas language skills decline during cognitive deficits, receptivity to music remains until the late phases of the disease. Since the 1990s, research on music's effect on cognitive deficiencies, particularly on patients with dementia, has been prolific.[11]

The London Study

In 2001, 20 patients suffering from dementia from the Department of Psychology at Surrey's University of London were subjected to autobiographical recall tasks (ability to recall or remember past events of one's life), both with and without background music, in a repeated-measures design. Familiar or novel music was played, with the pieces being matched on three affective scales. Autobiographical recall was found to be better for those facilitated by music, as opposed to those who had to recall in silence.[12]

UC-Davis Study

Sometime in 2009, more significant research in the domain of autobiographical recall came from Prof. Petr Janata, associate professor of psychology at the UC Davis Center for Mind and Brain. Not surprisingly, he targeted the same region in the brain that has been the darling of all studies concerning meditation, stress and Alzheimer's: the medial prefrontal cortex (MPFC).

---

[11]Gilbertson, Simon K., and David Aldridge, 'Searching PubMed/MEDLINE, Ingenta, and the Music Therapy World Journal Index for Articles Published in the Journal of Music Therapy', *Journal of Music Therapy*, Vol. 40, No. 4, 2003, pp. 324–44, http://tinyurl.com/288ffcmn. Accessed on 12 December 2023.

[12]Foster, N. A., and E.R. Valentine, 'The Effect of Concurrent Music on Autobiographical Recall in Dementia Clients' *Musicae Scientiae*, Vol. 2, No. 2, 1998, pp. 143–55.

Prof. Janata demonstrated the sterling role of the MPFC as the cradle of an association between the features of the music heard and autobiographical memories and emotions. Evidence also indicated that the strong recruitment of allied brain networks occurs during the reliving process of music-evoked autobiographical memories (MEAMs).[13]

In this study, 13 UC-Davis undergraduates (11 females and two males, in the age range of 18 to 22) listened to 30 excerpts presented across two scanning runs of 15 songs each, with each song lasting about 30 seconds. For each of these undergraduates, 30 stimuli were randomly selected from the Billboard Top 100 Pop and R&B (rhythm and blue: a general term for all African–American music) charts for the years when they were between seven to 19 years of age. Immediately after hearing the excerpts, the individuals were seated in front of a computer in a quiet room and instructed to complete a survey about their episodic memories of the songs they had signalled as autobiographically prominent. Along with the post-scan memory test and assay of the content, each individual underwent an MRI to track and correlate relevant activities in the brain.

Running through the responses, Prof. Janata observed strong associations between autobiographical prominence and memories thick with emotions and vivid remembrances. On an average, each participant recognized about 17 of the 30 excerpts, and of these, 13 carried moderate or strong associations with an autobiographical memory.

The MRI images were equally fascinating. They showed that the degree of autobiographical prominence had remarkable correlation and correspondence with the amount of activity in the dorsal part of the MPFC—the exact area where Alzheimer's causes damage.

---

[13]Janata, P., 'The Neural Architecture of Music-Evoked Autobiographical Memories', *Cerebral Cortex*, Vol. 19, No. 11, 2009, pp. 2579–94.

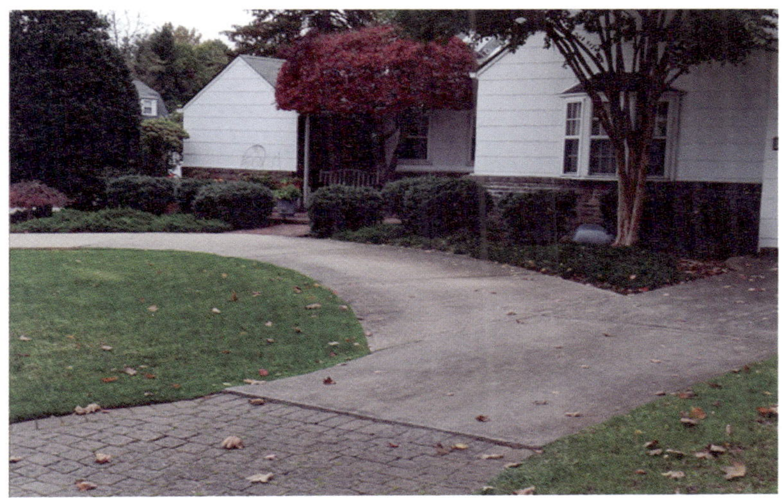

Closed, loopy and interconnected pathways, convenient for walks without losing the way

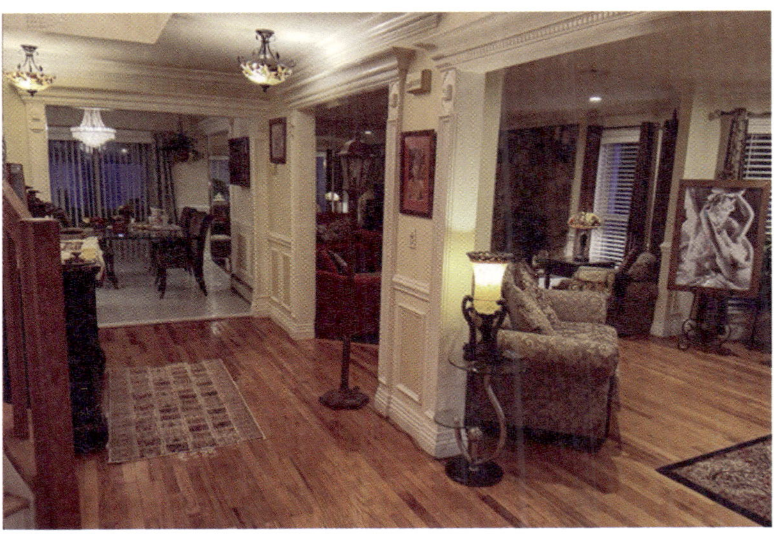

Non-institutional, homely set-up with open floor pattern convenient for Alzheimer's patients to ambulate. As can be seen, dining space is visible and hence accessible from all quarters.

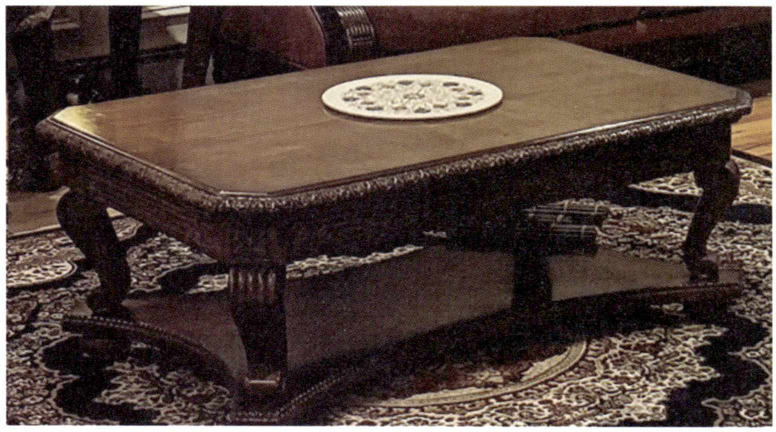

Furniture prototype: Table with round curves as opposed to sharp edges, with non-obstructive objects on table top

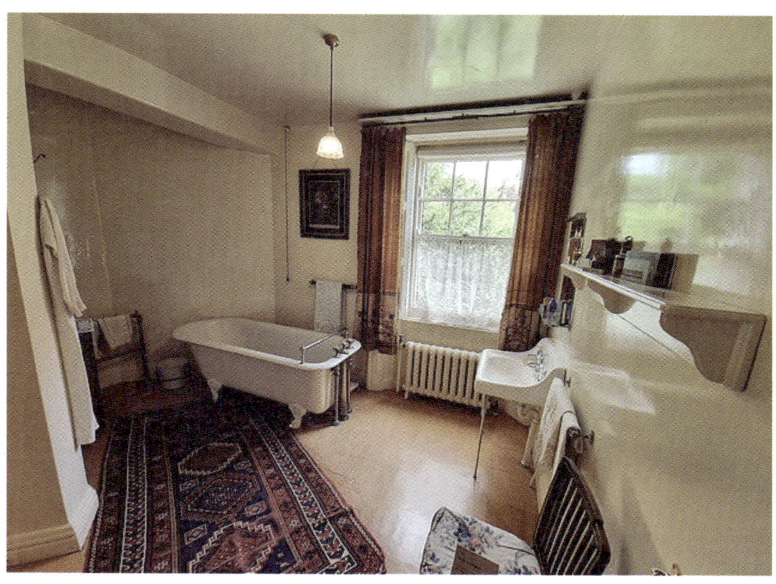

East accessibility and visibility of a bathroom with all amenities

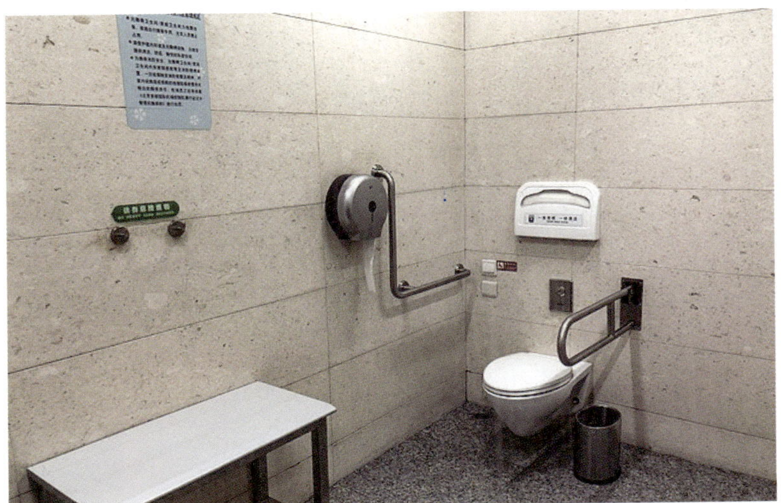

Commode with railing on both sides to facilitate better grip

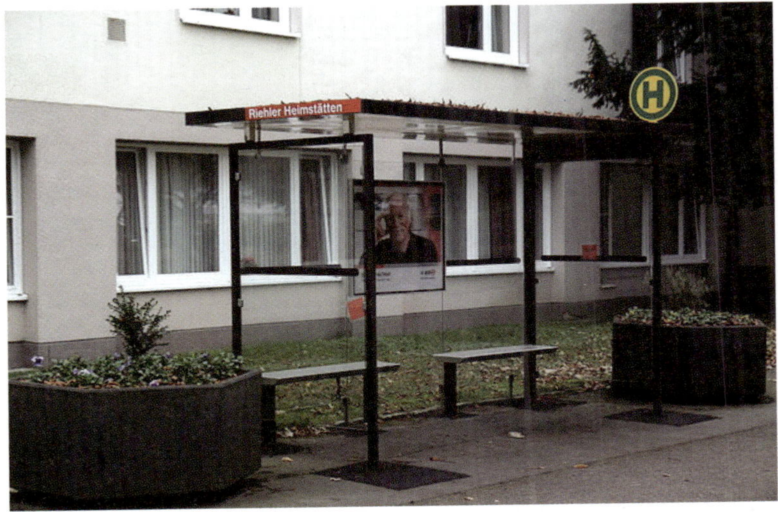

A bus stop in Riehler Heimstätten, a nursing home in Germany. No bus ever stops here, as it was installed solely as a novel therapeutic measure for dementia patients. It became a proven way to curb wandering traits seen in Alzheimer's patients.

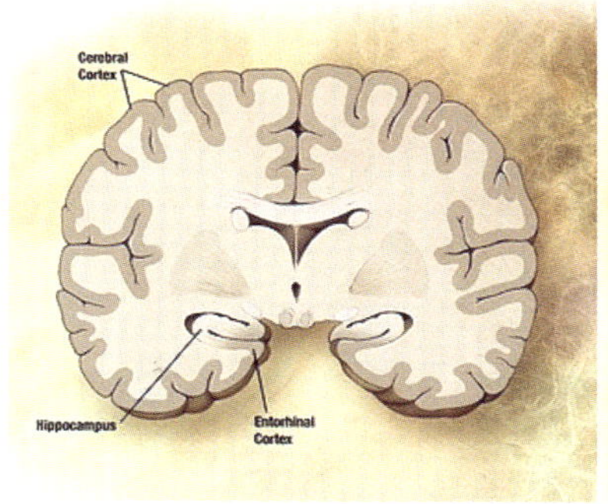

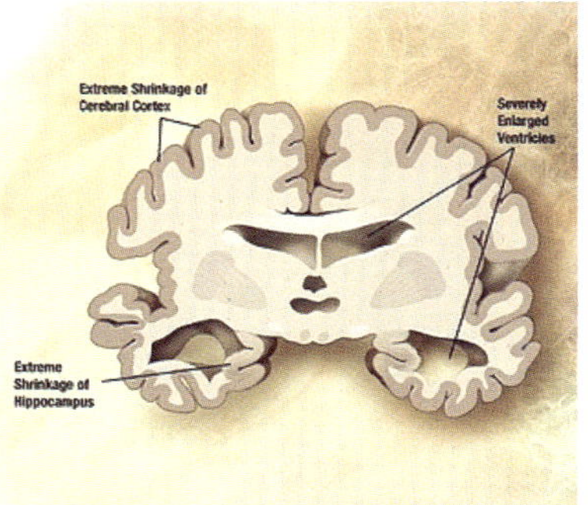

Generalized shrinkage of an Alzheimer's-affected brain

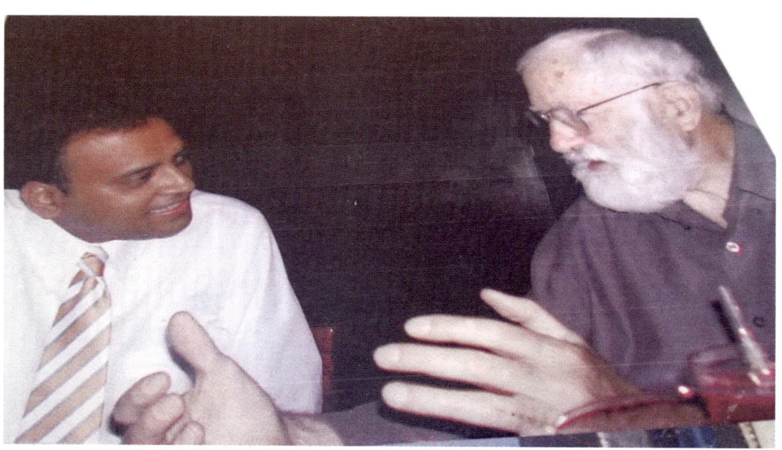

My interactions with Berkeley University neuroscientist Walter Freeman, MD, great grandson of Civil War surgeon, William Keen, United States' first brain surgeon. Freeman is one of the founders of computational neuroscience.

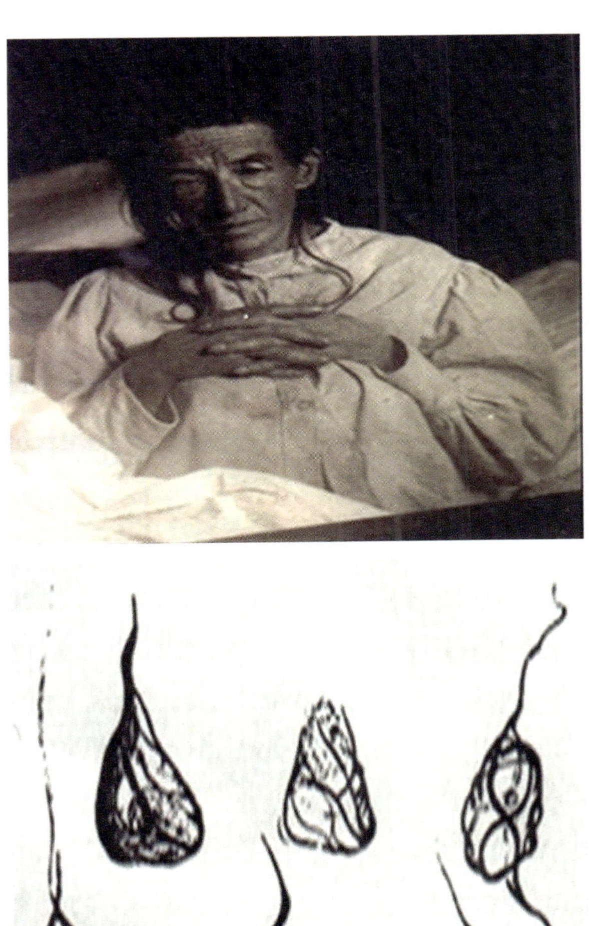

Auguste Deter, the first patient of Alois Alzheimer, and original drawings of Tau fibrils (tangled proteins in the brain, found in Alzheimer's and many other neurodegenerative diseases). Figures taken from the book *Alzheimer: 100 Years and Beyond*

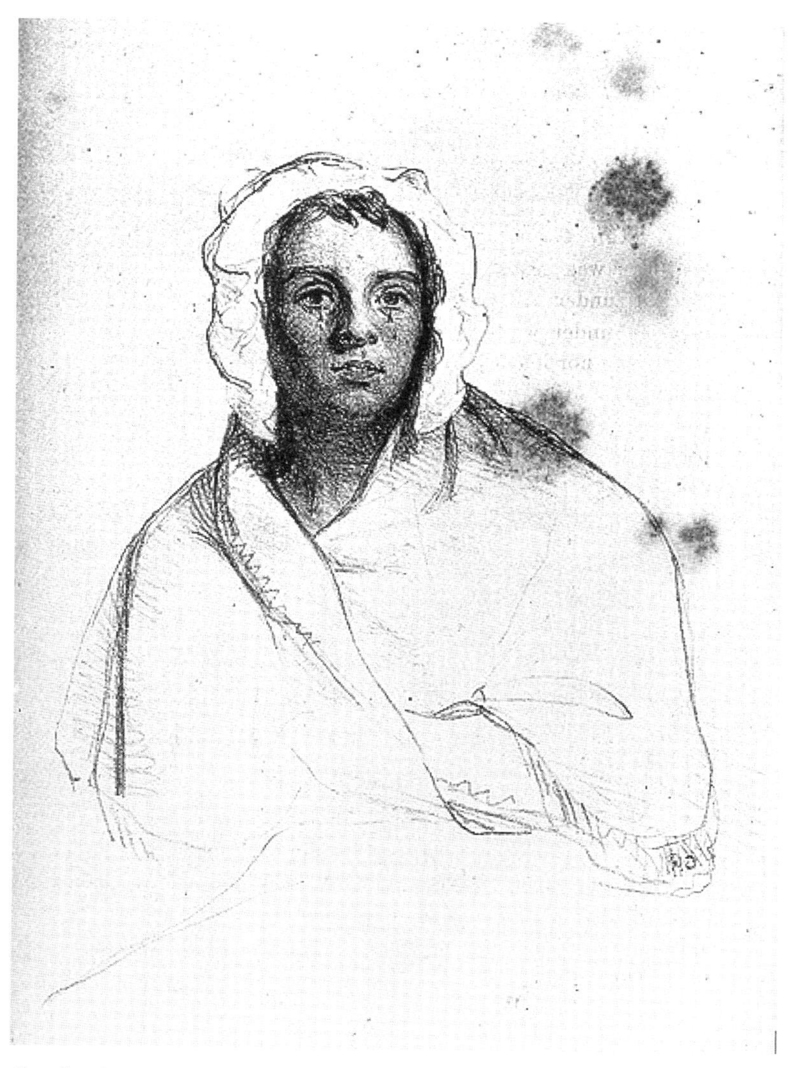

Sketch of a 20-year-young girl diagnosed with acute dementia at Bethlehem Hospital, circa 1848

Straßburg. Redner gedenkt in warmen und anerkennenden Worten des verstorbenen Psychiaters Prof. Dr. *Karl Fürstner* und gibt einen Überblick über das Leben und die wissenschaftlichen Verdienste und Arbeiten des Verstorbenen. Die Versammelten erheben sich zum ehrenden Andenken *Fürstners* von ihren Sitzen. *Kreuser*-Winnental berichtet über die an Geh. Rat *Ludwig*-Heppenheim zur Feier seines 80. Geburtstages eingereichte Glückwunschadresse und die Danksagung des Jubilars.

Vorträge.

1. *Bürker*-Tübingen: Zur Thermodynamik des Muskels.

Die dynamischen und elektrischen Verhältnisse der Muskelmaschine sind Gegenstand vielfältiger Untersuchungen gewesen. Zur genaueren Analyse der Wirkungsweise einer Maschine genügt aber nicht die Kenntnis ihres dynamischen Effektes, noch weniger die des nebenher auftretenden elektrischen, es muß hierzu vielmehr ermittelt werden: wieviel Brennmaterial wendet die Muskelmaschine auf und wieviel nutzbringende Arbeit leistet sie dabei? mit andern Worten: es muß bekannt sein der thermische Wirkungsgrad, die indizierte und die effektive Leistung.

Solche Untersuchungen ermöglicht wenigstens an Kaltblütermuskeln die thermodynamische Methodik. Mit ihrer Hülfe wurde ermittelt, daß die Muskelmaschine unter den verschiedenen äußeren und inneren Einflüssen, wie sie die verschiedene Jahreszeit mit sich bringt, über gesetzmäßig verschiedene Mengen von Brennmaterial verfügt und dieses auch in den einzelnen Jahreszeiten in verschiedener Weise verwertet, daß die weiblichen Froschmuskeln in der Laichzeit reich an Brennmaterial und daher sehr leistungsfähig sind, daß Krötenmuskeln unter sonst gleichen Bedingungen zur Ermöglichung einer maximalen Zuckung nur halb so viel Energie aufwenden und Arbeit leisten als Froschmuskeln, daß das Adduktorenpräparat mit halb so viel Brennmaterial doppelt soviel Arbeit zu leisten vermag als das Gastrocnemiuspräparat, was außerordentlich auffallend erscheint, daß es eine Heizung des Muskels auf Nervenreiz hin, ohne daß es zu einer Kontraktion kommt, nicht gibt, daß es bezüglich des Energieaufwandes gleichgültig ist, ob direkt oder indirekt gereizt wird, falls nur die Arbeitsleistung gleich groß ausfällt, daß bei einer Muskelzuckung der Zug des angehängten Gewichtes nicht nur im Stadium der steigenden Energie, sondern auch in dem der sinkenden Energie exothermische Prozesse, wenn auch in geringerem Maße, auslöst.

(Eigenbericht).

Keine Diskussion.

2. *Alzheimer*-München: Über eine eigenartige Erkrankung der Hirnrinde.

A. berichtet über einen Krankheitsfall, der in der Irrenanstalt in Frankfurt a. M. beobachtet und dessen Centralnervensystem ihm von Herrn Direktor Sioli zur Untersuchung überlassen wurde.

First documented description of Azheimer's dementia by Dr Alois Alzheimer in 1906

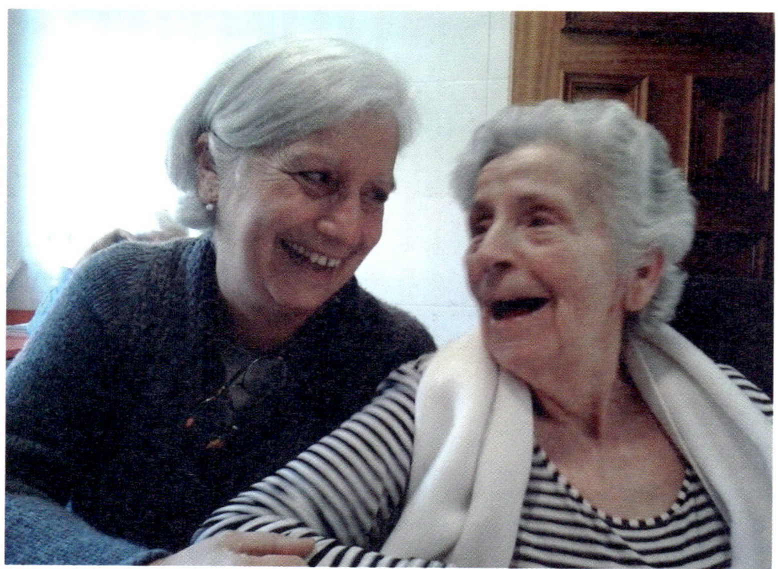

In the journey of looking after an Alzheimer's patient, their loved one also needs to be looked after. Care is sacrosanct for both.

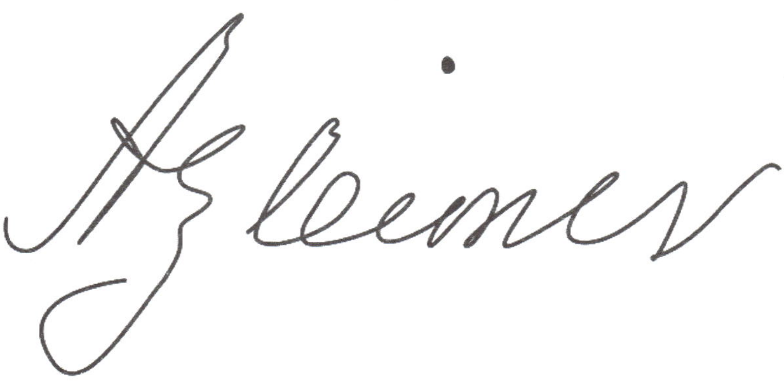

Signature of Alois Alzheimer, 1915

From here, an extraordinary venture followed. With a firmly held hypothesis that the MPFC held music and memory together, Prof. Janata and his research team actually tracked the inner trajectory of a rendition or score heard as it meandered across the 24 major and minor keys that are the foundation of Western tonal music.

They tracked the tonal progressions with sequential brain scans, and to their delight, the regions of the brain that retrieved memories fell along the same track of the tonal progressions. In fact, the stronger the autobiographical memory, the greater the tracking activity.

The Finnish Study

Two years later, Vinoo Alluri and her colleagues from the Finnish Center of Excellence at the University of Jyväskylä in Finland, took a step beyond the work of Prof. Janata.[14] They dived more deeply into the subtle aspects of a musical rendition, including rhythm, tonality and timbre, and correlated them with the areas of the brain affiliated and responsible for the processing of the same. In this logical and intuitive study, they found a wide network of brain structures to be involved and activated during music listening, including, but not limited to, cognitive areas of the cerebellum, cortical and subcortical areas.

According to Prof. Petri Toiviainen, one of the collaborators in the research, their results show how different musical features activate emotional, motor and creative areas of the brain. He believes that their method provides more reliable knowledge about music processing in the brain than the more conventional methods.

Why did Prof. Toiviainen think theirs was a unique endeavour? It was so because this was the first time such a study was conducted

[14]Alluri, Vinoo, et al., 'Large-Scale Brain Networks Emerge from Dynamic Processing of Musical Timbre, Key and Rhythm', *NeuroImage*, Vol. 59, No. 4, 2012, pp. 3677–89.

using real music to replace the artificially constructed, music-like stimuli that had been used in past studies. To that end, participants listened to a piece of a modern Argentinian tango, while researchers analysed the musical content of the piece, showing how its rhythmic, tonal and timbral components evolved over time. They then compared the brain's responses and the musical features.

The results were a testimony to the diversity and depth of music in its relationship with our brain. Listening to music, as shown in the study, recruits not only auditory areas of the brain but also a wider network of areas. While the motor area of the brain processed the musical pulse, authenticating the idea that music and movement are entwined, rhythm and tonality involved the limbic area, also known as an emotional hot spot.

As we realize now, the hub at the prefrontal cortex and the promises of autobiographical memory recovered by music have become a passionate pilgrimage for researchers.

An Australian Study

Two years later, in 2013, scientists Amee Baird and Séverine Samson from the University of Newcastle in Australia, focussed on their study regarding patients with severe acquired brain injury (ABI).[15] Their daring goal was to prove that popular music could evoke autobiographical memories. Accordingly, five ABI patients, along with matched controls, listened to extracts from Billboard's Top 100. The study line recalled Prof. Janata's experimental approach of playing songs having a nostalgic value. This time, however, the renditions were taken from the whole of the patients' life span, starting from the age of five, and familiarity was sought through a questionnaire, Autobiographical Memory

[15]Baird, A., and S. Samson, 'Music Evoked Autobiographical Memory After Severe Acquired Brain Injury: Preliminary Findings From a Case Series', *Neuropsychological Rehabilitation*, Vol. 24, No. 1, 2014, pp. 125–43.

Interview (AMI) and neuropsychological assessment. Invariably, the songs that aroused memory buried after the brain injury were found to be more familiar and more well-liked than songs that failed to trigger a positive response.

MUSIC AND ALZHEIMER'S: LET'S GET TO THE POINT

As recently as 2016, José Carlos Millán Calenti, along with his colleagues from the Gerontology Research Group, Department of Medicine, at the Universidade da Coruña, in Spain, conducted a systematic review of randomized controlled trials (RCTs), focussing on the non-pharmacological management of agitation, specifically of Alzheimer's patients, with the aim of making evidence-based recommendations about the use of specific intervention strategies. Of all the other non-pharmacological methods assessed—including cognitive stimulation/training, behavioural interventions, physical exercise, therapeutic touch, aromatherapy and bright light therapy—music therapy stood out as one of the most promising and profound.[16]

The results were particularly visible when the intervention was geared specifically for a particular individual. In other words, maximum benefit was obtained when music that categorically related to evoking positive memories *unique* to a patient was played, opposed to any generic versions for the entire group in context. Equally strong results were obtained when the music was interactive, beckoning active participation with clapping, singing and dancing.

The researchers used a standard and popular scale to assess agitation: the BEHAVE-AD. It covers behavioural symptoms in seven categories: paranoid and delusional ideations; hallucinations;

[16]Millán-Calenti, José Carlos, et al., 'Optimal Non-pharmacological Management of Agitation in Alzheimer's Disease: Challenges and Solutions', *Clinical Interventions in Aging*, Vol. 11, 2016, pp. 175–84.

activity disturbances; aggressiveness; diurnal rhythm disturbances; affective disturbances; and anxieties and phobias (a higher score indicates more severity). The researchers probed the long-term effects of passive (listening to music from a CD player) or interactive (including clapping, singing and dancing) music therapy, lasting for 10 weeks.

A higher, long-term reduction was observed in behavioural symptoms in the interactive music group, compared with the passive music group and no-music control group, which received the usual care rendered.

The music facilitators included two music therapists, four occupational therapists and six nurses. Each intervention was performed once a week and lasted 30 minutes. Individualized music was selected, related to specific positive memories for each participant.

The results were gratifying but not surprising, as the scores of five items of the BEHAVE-AD—paranoid and delusional ideations, activity disturbances, aggressiveness, affective disturbances, and anxieties and phobias—were significantly reduced in the group with interactive music.

How long did these positive benefits sustain? Sure enough, as this experiment showed, the effects on decreasing agitation did not last long, with benefits dwindling progressively and eventually disappearing, after three weeks from the cessation of the interventions.

What does all this indicate? It simply shows that the effects are contingent on the active involvement of the patients concerned—just like, we may add, the good effects of a company-driven drug. We scientists walk the same paths here, except in the glorious differences relating to adverse effects and tolerance—both of which are the perilous effects of a prescribed pill.

These results also revisit a fundamental concept of music therapy, or for that matter, any non-pharmacological therapy. When it comes to the treatment or management of cognitive disorders, the approach needs to be patient-centric. We remind ourselves again and again that every Alzheimer's disease is different, just as every individual is unique.

Intriguingly, more than MDs, nurses have championed the use of music therapy as an indispensable intervention for patients with dementia and allied cognitive disorders. In an article, author H. Ragneskog, among others, described the reactions of five patients with dementia to three different types of music during dinner. The entire episode was filmed. One of the study's restless patients showed decreasing agitation, and the other patient actually fed himself more than usual, while in general, all patients preferred to spend more time on the dinner table as the music lingered.[17]

These reactions hit the very core of medical research—in terms of incorporating holistic options within the framework of standard innovations. The situation only became stickier when it approached the idea of music as therapy.

As I have hinted earlier, the problem lies in our mindset. It is useless to force down one's throat the trademark trials and tribulations to which a drug is subjected, for music is *not* a drug. It is an internal feeling, a subjective choice, a mood elevator that is at once personal and momentary. I say momentary only because the same piece of music that comes as rejuvenating, refreshing and reviving can turn passé, dispensable and ordinary at another time of day or in another mood. In other words, we are caught between 'music over mind' versus 'mind over music'. While certain music has been shown to have the capability of taming the untamed, for most individuals, receptivity of the mind takes precedence over music, per se. We go overboard trying to demonstrate the benefits of music without having

---

[17]Ragneskog, H., et al., 'Individualized Music Played for Agitated Patients with Dementia: Analysis of Video-Recorded Sessions', *International Journal of Nursing Practice*, 2001, Vol. 7, pp. 146–55.

the knowledge or understanding of how it actually works and achieves its outcomes.

'But it works!' Andrew DeNicola bellowed to me when I asked him about the benefits of music. Affiliated for more than 30 years with J.P. Steven High School in Edison, New Jersey, DeNicola received a nomination for a Grammy Award as a music teacher.

'How do you think music helps your students, or yourself, for that matter?' I asked, sitting in his office with him, while his students rehearsed.

'Simply put, it relieves the stress,' he said. 'I see these students. Their nerves are shot. But when they come to me, and when they play with me, they are instantly calmed. Something happens. I don't know what.'

Let me swing back to some immensely successful stories and drive home our musical pledge.

From Coma to Home: The Fascinating Case of Dawn Shilling

Dawn Shilling was a 22-year-old patient who was admitted to our hospital in a state of complete unresponsiveness, due to a drug overdose after a fight with her boyfriend. The Glasgow Coma Scale, the standard neurological scale to assess a patient's conscious state, read 5 out of 12. Neurologists ordered an MRI of her head, which showed features suggesting anoxic encephalopathy. She remained bed-bound, on mechanical ventilation and essential comfort medicines. With no meaningful expectations, our hospital neurologist called her family members to explain the future course of action. The idea was to get her family's opinion for either continued therapy or withdrawal of active care. Accordingly, the Bioethics Committee was summoned.

It was explained in painful detail how Dawn would remain bed-ridden and tied to ventilation with little to no to chance of meaningful recovery. All family members, except John, her father, agreed to the futility of further care. John was a retired construction worker who had bent over backwards to raise his children. After his wife had died of a sudden stroke, his daughter was all he lived for, and he refused to budge, despite social workers, clinicians and other family members trying to convince him.

Active management continued, despite the administrative eyebrows that continued to be raised with each passing day. I shifted Dawn to a quieter room, away from the hustle and bustle of the central nursing station. I saw no reason for meaningless weather channels and TV soap operas in her room and recommended Gospel music, much to the delight of her father, who was a religious man and remained steadfast day and night by her bedside, half-reclined on an armchair. I told him to talk and read scriptures to Dawn as if she was listening. He did so with unfailing devotion.

Nothing happened and nothing moved. We maintained the ventilation management, the PEG (percutaneous endoscopic gastrostomy) tube feeding, the IV fluids and the Gospel music. One day, John called me late one evening, his voice trembling.

'I think I saw Dawn's eyes roll over. And her fingers trembled. Maybe she is communicating?'

I did not have the heart to tell him that those could be natural movements, periodic and involuntary reflexes. The following morning, on my rounds with my residents, I tried something different. I lowered my voice, and slid my ungloved index finger into Dawn's half-crumpled palm and whispered to her, 'If you can hear me, Dawn, squeeze my finger.'

After what seemed like forever, Dawn's fingers quivered, subtle and slight, almost in protest. I looked up at John, who stood at the other end of the bed, his lips trembling, his eyes a raging river of tears. I knew the battle was far from over. I wanted nothing to change, I wanted traditional medicine to stay back, with gospel and John sustaining the moment.

Dawn recovered, muscle by muscle, motion by motion. One

morning, she moved her eyes. One afternoon, she consumed her first liquid diet in two months. A month later, she was wheeled out of Room No. 516, followed by 20 joyous family members.

Did Dawn recover naturally? Was she an exception to the rule? Did John's soothing words, day in and day out, unplug Dawn's clogged brain? Did the relentless gospel music awaken her comatose brain?

We do not have answers to any of these questions. We do know that Dawn turned around—against all medical dictates. We do know that other than ventilation management and PEG tube feeding, no other medical intervention was offered. And we know that the room was flooded with music of the most profound depth and demeanour.

We will do well to keep our perspectives right here. The worst we can do is place Dawn's personal experience among other comatose patients, play the gospel music and search for statistical significance.

We over-glorify facts and figures while the magic of personal healing gets demonized as exceptional and coincidental. More objectively, music becomes that unseen bridge across which memories, dead and defunct, become recollections, viable and visible.

Music from Oliver Sacks, the Poet Laureate of Medicine

I will end this discussion on music therapy with Oliver Sacks, one of the rare neurologists who did not let knowledge muffle the intuitive insight that can traverse the obvious. In his descriptions of his experiences with Parkinson's patients, both personal and poignant, he highlighted the absolute importance of music as a healing companion.

Several examples come out of Sacks' endless experiences: a woman with advanced Alzheimer's who was still able to memorize intricate and newly learned piano compositions; a musician grounded with Alzheimer's who could actually play and record at a higher level than before; and an elderly gentleman who knew baritone parts to a cappella songs from memory but could not otherwise say who he was.

Dr Sacks echoed the essences of previous experiments: familiar and comforting music is more likely to evoke lost memories of an individual suffering from dementia. He went a step further and recommended 'movement' in group therapy. According to him, dance, because it is multi-modal, becomes an effective tool to infuse animation in patients who are sunk in the doldrums. Even drum circles as a possible therapy carry promise because they call upon 'very fundamental, subcortical levels of the brain'.[18]

Along with all my colleagues, I cannot, in any rational view, call music a cure for Alzheimer's. It is irrational to believe that it will untangle the amyloid plugs. Yet, a profound truth remains: music moves every soul. Sometimes, it simmers and sometimes, it stirs. It is there, though, always in the vast and deep reservoir of our minds. To sufferers, it offers a timeless moment to recover lost selves. To caregivers, it opens a rare window to watch their loved ones return.

When Bidisha's Mother Turned the Clock Back with Music

I will end with Bidisha's mother. In my long medical career, spanning decades and oceans, I have seldom come across such great gratification within such a short period of time.

I was in her sprawling Navi Mumbai flat, when Bidisha mentioned about her mother sunk in Alzheimer's. Her natural eloquence did not betray any hidden feelings. As the conversation went deeper, I learnt that her mother was an exquisite Rabindra Sangeet singer under the tutelage of Debabrata Biswas, a legendary

---

[18]Bruchhage, Murie M.K., et al., 'Drum Training Induces Long-Term Plasticity in the Cerebellum and Connected Cortical Thickness', *Scientific Reports*, 2020, https://tinyurl.com/rjr2ckmc. Accessed on 5 December 2023.

exponent of that genre of music.

'Does she sing now?' I had asked

'Now? She hardly speaks.' Bidisha's answer was flat.

'Does she listen to her favourite compositions?'

'Once in a while.'

'Why don't you make her listen like a ritual? Flood her room with Rabindra Sangeet!' I couldn't conceal my enthusiasm.

Hardly a month later, I received a call from Bidisha. She was screaming over the phone, 'My mom is singing. She looks full of life when singing!'

FIVE

WHEN MEDICINE IS NOT *JUST* ABOUT PRESCRIPTIONS

'I don't do drugs. I am drugs.'

—Salvador Dali, Spanish artist

Coming from a physician who encourages and endorses the appropriate use of over-the-counter drugs and routinely prescribes medications, including controlled substances, this chapter may appear paradoxical. To the millions who otherwise would have been crushed under the boots of infectious and non-infectious diseases, this might even seem blasphemous. It is not my intention to castigate the same drugs that human lives and my academic expertise depend on. Neither should the following pages be viewed as the retreating steps of a physician close to retirement from active practice. I am not a leader of a vanguard or a whistle-blower.

For the last 30 years, I have practised clinical medicine, which rests on a triad of diagnosis, treatment and prevention. Prescription and non-prescription drugs are legitimate and undisputed fulcrums of many cures. Yet, from this very throne of power brews a resistance in the making, and like a landmine at every bend, this resistance stems from the way we practise patient care today.

To be specific, the insurmountable challenge comes from the overuse of drugs. Like any human trait that is indulged once it promises and promotes happiness, we also overexercise our power to control and conquer. And like any power-hungry soul, we bleed from the very sword we create to protect and preserve. History will explain our present and hopefully guide our future.

DRUGS THAT CAN CAUSE DEMENTIA

There are over-the-counter popularly used drugs that actually run the risk of causing dementia. This is a growing expansive list, and only time will tell how many more will jump on the bandwagon in near future.

Anticholinergics

Although not conclusive, studies show that these inhibitors of acetylcholine (a chemical substance necessary for memory and traditionally found to be low in Alzheimer's patients) have been linked with growing dementia. The fact that some of these, called antihistamines, are commonly found over the counter and are used for common cold make matters leery.[1] Also included in this category are some examples of antidepressants and drugs used for Irritable Bowel Syndrome.

Proton Pump Inhibitors

It may not be an exaggeration to say that every second or third individual in India and across the globe uses this class of medication. Popularly called omeprazole, pantoprazole and lansoprazole, these are literally swallowed like candies. Recent studies showing their associations with dementia has set alarms in the medical fraternity.[2]

---

[1]Gray S.L., et al., 'Cumulative Use of Strong Anticholinergics and Incident Dementia: A Prospective Cohort Study', *JAMA Internal Medicine*, Vol. 175, No. 3, 2015, pp. 401–07.

[2]Gomm, W., et al., 'Association of Proton Pump Inhibitors with Risk of Dementia: A Pharmacoepidemiological Claims Data Analysis', *JAMA Neurology*, Vol. 73, No. 4, 2016, pp. 410-6.

Pain Medications

Another class of medications, used and prescribed at will, are the pain medications, including not just the heavyweights like morphine but the easily accessible ones like ibuprofen and naproxen.[3] Studies increasingly show their link with dementia.

Benzodiazepine Drugs

For those who are sleepless even after midnight, these class of drugs are their guardian angels. Yet, lorazepam, diazepam and alprazolam have always been held with caution by doctors, for long-time users have reported frequent falling, confusion, drowsiness and over-all sluggish behaviour. Now, with studies indicating its possible association with dementia, the circle of fear seems complete.[4]

ALZHEIMER'S AND DRUGS: HOW THEY WORK, WHY THEY DON'T

Regarding Alzheimer's, we are every bit like the five wise but blind men who are observing different parts of an elephant and generating generous opinions of what it is. The diverse and thoroughly unrelated theories about the genesis of Alzheimer's feel as discrete as the tusk, trunk, tail, teeth and belly of the animal. Among the countless theories trying to rationalize the aberration of the human mind, some verge on the romantic while others are worse than fanatic. However, two theories stand out as plausible.

---

[3]Dublin, S., et al., 'Prescription Opioids and Risk of Dementia or Cognitive Decline: A Prospective Cohort Study', *Journal of the American Geriatrics Society*, Vol. 63, No. 8, 2015, pp. 1519–26.

[4]Lucchetta, R.C., Barbara Paes Miglioli da Mata and Patricia de Carvalho Mastroianni, 'Association between Development of Dementia and Use of Benzodiazepines: A Systematic Review and Meta-Analysis', *Pharmacotherapy*, Vol. 38, No. 10, 2018, pp. 1010–20.

They do not define the disease—far from it—but they do unearth fractions of milestones in the pathology of its events.

As scientists always do, they blaze a trail as they follow the exact path of a progression of a disease. From antihypertensive drugs for high blood pressure to chemotherapy for cancer, this approach remains set in stone. This also applies to drugs for Alzheimer's. But given that the major road leading to Alzheimer's is yet undiscovered, no drugs can specifically blaze that trail.

Donepezil

To start with, scientists discovered that patients with Alzheimer's have a decrease in acetylcholine synthesis (an excitatory substance that carries message from the brain to our body), which they believed was one of the prime mechanisms underlying the functional wreck of the mind. True to the scientific spirit, scientists engineered inhibitors of these excitatory substances.

Pfizer, the multibillion-dollar company, rolled out donepezil. The drug was primarily researched at Esai, a Japanese pharmaceutical company headquartered in Tokyo, in 1983, under the supervision of Hachiro Sugimoto, a Japanese chemist and pharmacologist. In 1996, with US Food and Drug Administration approval under its belt, Pfizer rolled it out as aricept. The drug soon became the global star invading virtually every Alzheimer's mind with unrestricted entry. In an exciting 24-week-double-blind study that entailed blinding both the examiners and the subjects of the study to be unaware of the drug being tested, significant improvement was seen, compared to the control groups.[5]

The crash came soon after. Following the initial 24-week study, researchers conducted the all-important six-week placebo washout study (the period allowed for all of the administered

[5]Shigeta, M., and A. Homma, 'Donepezil for Alzheimer's Disease: Pharmacodynamic, Pharmacokinetic, and Clinical Profiles', *CNS Drug Reviews*, Vol. 7, No. 4, 2001, pp. 353–68.

drugs to be eliminated from the body) to examine whether donepezil had any disease-modifying activity. The results were horrific. The earlier improvements detected on cognitive measures had been completely erased, strongly suggesting that the drug did not affect the underlying course of the disease. Even worse, with no significant differences in global functioning, treatment-emergent adverse effects were more frequently observed in the higher-dose group. Nausea, vomiting, diarrhoea, decreased heart rate and, at times, brief unconsciousness, concluded this chapter of misery.

Rivastigmine

Undeterred by the results of donepezil, Novartis Pharmaceuticals manufactured rivastigmine, a drug that harboured similar mechanism of action. Initially developed by Marta Weinstock-Rosin of the Department of Pharmacology at the Hebrew University of Jerusalem, the drug became available in liquid and capsule formulations in 1997. It demonstrated the same efficacies and adverse effects as its predecessor.[6]

Scientists then tried something novel. In 2007, they manufactured a transdermal patch form of the drug to minimize the gastrointestinal side effects of nausea, vomiting and diarrhoea. Yet, when it came to long-term benefits, the results were equally inconclusive.

Galantamine

Galantamine came next. Formally released in 2001, it came nearly 50 years after Soviet pharmacologists M.D. Mashkovsky and R.P. Kruglikova-Lvova had worked on the memory enhancing properties of acetylcholine, a substance found in the brain. Previously called reminyl and now razadyne, the drug had similar

---

[6]Figiel, Gary, and Carl Sadowsky, 'A Systematic Review of the Effectiveness of Rivastigmine for the Treatment of Behavioral Disturbances in Dementia and Other Neurological Disorders', *Current Medical Research and Opinion*, Vol. 24, No. 1, 2008, pp. 157–66.

effects but stole the limelight for a different reason. One particular study found that it actually increased mortality when given to patients with mild cognitive impairment.[7]

With lesser adverse effects and comparable benefits, donepezil emerged as the leading product, but nursing home patients who had advanced Alzheimer's dementia provided no conclusive data, showing comprehensive benefit. Even for patients with mild cognitive impairment, considered possible precursors of Alzheimer's, none of these drugs offered an olive branch.

Therein lies the overarching tragedy.

Demonstrating short-term cognitive benefits without the power of prevention or cure, these drugs become a cruel tease for the sufferer. Yet, out of habit, and perhaps motivated by guilt, we continue to dispense these drugs that seem to momentarily enhance our memory and thought process.

Memantine

With memantine, scientists took another route. Glutamate was discovered in the early 1960s as another excitatory substance found in the hippocampus area of the brain, the prime location for memory. It was found to activate a receptor (a molecule inside or on the surface of a cell that receives and binds with a substance) that is responsible for memory and learning. As too much excitation is harmful for the nerves, the search was on to find a drug to oppose the excessive excitation. As a receptor antagonist, memantine fit the bill perfectly. Haughtily termed a 'neuroprotective' in areas of memory and learning, it entered the market under the brand name Namenda.[8]

---

[7]Hager, Klaus, et al., 'Effects of Galantamine in a 2-Year, Randomized, Placebo-Controlled Study in Alzheimer's Disease', *Neuropsychiatric Disease and Treatment*, Vol. 10, 2014, pp. 391–401.

[8]Thomas, Stuart J., George G. Grossberg, 'Memantine: A Review of Studies into Its Safety and Efficacy in Treating Alzheimer's Disease and Other Dementias', *Clinical Interventions in Aging*, Vol. 4, 2009, pp. 367–77.

Before it was known as a neuroprotective agent, memantine was touted as an antidiabetic agent and released into society by Eli Lilly and Company back in 1968. Found to be useless, it was sent back to the drawing board. More than 20 years later, the Merz Company from Germany found its neuroprotective effects and sent it back into circulation. This time, it was meant to save the brain from dementia. It took less than a decade for the US-based Forest Laboratories to shake hands with Merz, nickname it Namenda, and launch it into a society that was starving for another miracle drug.

Needless to say, namenda did little to cure the demented brain. There was little, if any, evidence that patients with milder Alzheimer's dementia would benefit from this drug. Instead, a different set of adverse effects arose. With dizziness as its primary disturbing effect, the drug has been reported to cause confusion, hallucination and, in some cases, agitation and delusional behaviours in patients with Alzheimer's.

A 2008 systemic review by experts concluded, 'Memantine has been shown to improve cognition and global assessment of dementia, but with small effects that are not of clear clinical significance; improvement in quality of life and other domains are suggested but not proven.'[9]

Unanswered questions continued to pour in: 'Will long-term treatment benefit those with mild AD?', 'Is it truly neuroprotective?', 'How will that be manifested?'

Almost all experts concurred that decisions to treat with Namenda are strictly to be determined on an individual basis, dependent on the physician, patient, or family choice, and must consider drug tolerability and cost. Unfortunately, this requires a perfect balancing act on a beam that does not actually exist.

---

[9]McShane, Rupert, et al., 'Memantine for Dementia', *The Cochrane Database of Systematic Reviews,* Vol. 3, No, 3, 2019.

Lecanemab

The last to enter the arena is lecanemab, a drug that removes a toxic protein from the brain. The results are promising, but again, marginal and underwhelming.[10]

In a market that is uncertain and volatile, it is natural to entertain all that a fertile mind can imagine. Endless cures and prevention strategies of Alzheimer's dementia scurry in and out, like rats in an abandoned building.

We stand today in a no-man's land, where overlapping diseases spew signs and symptoms for us to wash them away with buckets of pills. In between, patients remain inaccessible, captive in their own emotions.

WHEN BLIND DOCTORS TURN DRUG LORDS

While flipping through the chart of a new female patient, Susan, I gathered that she suffered from various psychiatric disorders. She had all of the patient's morbidities dated to the month. However, what emerged from her detailed notes was strange and disturbing. This is what the patient's past medical history looked like:

Time of Onset		**Diagnosis**
December 2001	:	Anxiety
July 2002	:	Bipolar Disorder
September 2004	:	Panic disorder
February 2006	:	Major Depression, Borderline Personality Disorder

While hypothetically possible, did Susan really have all these emotional challenges? Who was making these diagnoses? Was it a solitary, over-exuberant psychiatrist? Even more alarming was the endless list of medications she was subjected to. For

[10]Dyck, Christopher H. van, et al., 'Lecanemab in Early Alzheimer's Disease', *The New England Journal of Medicine*, Vol. 388, No. 1, 2023, pp. 9–21.

each diagnosis, she was given an antidote: an anxiolytic, an antipsychotic, a sedative and an antidepressant.

Susan refused to talk to me. She was determined not to disengage herself from her silent, unspoken cocoon. All my open-ended questions remained unanswered.

'Would you like to share anything with me?'

'Do you have family support?'

'Do you need any counseling?'

Instead, Susan stood up abruptly and blurted out, 'If you are not giving me the refills, I am getting out of here.'

'I will continue some of the medications,' I said, 'but before that we need to.' I started to reason with her but couldn't. She turned and stomped out in a flash.

Susan never came back. Three months later, she was brought to the emergency room with cardio-pulmonary arrest due to a possible heroin overdose. She died before she could be admitted.

MY FATHER-IN-LAW

My father-in-law, Prasenjit Chaudhuri, possessed a keen intellect, ferociously read all that fell under his eyelashes and revelled in arguments that leapt from philosophy to politics with a vivacious appetite. Health-wise, he lived a flawless life.

At the stroke of 80, he noticed a slowing of his gait. It was more of a shuffle, he thought. In the ensuing weeks, he had difficulty raising himself from his chair. He needed someone to pull him up each time he attempted to stand. His gait became unsteady. He preferred short steps, so as not to lean over. He felt weak and, in certain situations, even had a sense of freezing over. There was no tremor. The neurologist who examined him started him on levodopa/carbidopa, the undisputed healer of Parkinson's disease.

With no improvement seen from the pills, he panicked. Melancholy settled in. He turned inward. Words became scarcer and scarcer. Enter a psychiatrist. A rushed examination gave him

20 out of 30. Diagnosed with 'possible' Alzheimer's, he was put on donepezil, and, following close on its heels, an antidepressant. Nothing happened. He was estranged from the world. Another drug was prescribed, a benzodiazepine called lorazepam, to curb his growing anxiety.

Buffeted by quadruple 'mind-curing' medications, he oscillated from tears to anger to nothingness. The doctor recommended an institutional approach. A new set of doctors arrived with fresh diagnoses and medications. In a day or two, he started to hallucinate, first in bits and pieces, then in a continuous display of a fragmented mind, torn between images seen and imagined.

It became obvious that he was suffering from abrupt drug withdrawal. It was time to panic—this time for the doctors. They reintroduced lorazepam. Alzheimer's was ruled out. Donepezil was stopped. A touch of antidepressants remained.

An expressionless Mr Chaudhuri was sent home. No firm diagnosis could be established before he eventually breathed his last.

SIX

EAST PERCEIVED, WEST PURSUED: THE RISE OF HOLISTIC MEDICINE

'Oh, East is East, and West is West, and never the twain shall meet,
Till Earth and Sky stand presently at God's great Judgement Seat;
But there is neither East nor West, Border, nor Breed, nor Birth,
When two strong men stand face to face, though they come from the ends of the earth.'

—Rudyard Kipling, English novelist and poet

No words can transcend the prophetic thoughts of Rudyard Kipling as immortalized in 'The Ballad of East and West'. What the poet had conceptualized years ago is a present-day wondrous spectacle in the world of science and arts, where proposals from the East entice the West in a never-ending love affair.

MEDITATION UNDER THE MICROSCOPE

What has been found in test after test is that meditation achieves much more than external focus. The benefits affect the deepest centres of the brain, causing structural and even functional changes that can effectively keep Alzheimer's at bay. This is not just a feel-good but a scientifically measured fact.

Meditation has come a long way since its primordial moments in the deep recesses of a forest, where ancient sages practised this art as a way of life. From their teachings to the research-laden laboratories of Ivy League institutes, it has undertaken a groundbreaking journey, offering one blessing after another.

Let's take a look at the concepts, philosophies and benefits of each type of meditation.

Transcendental Meditation

In terms of how Transcendental Meditation (TM) arrests the development of Alzheimer's, we need to remind ourselves of two parallel events that accompany the disease.

First, Alzheimer's is not just about the sufferer forgetting things. An entire spectrum of emotions descends on those suffering from it. As we know and as discussed before, afflicted patients can harbour agitation, personality changes, severe depression, stress, an inability to execute complex functions and many other cognitive deficiencies. Each of these components serve to escalate the other.

Second, Alzheimer's is not a solitary disease. The whole family gets affected. The caregiver in particular—in most cases, spouses or children—suffer these pangs with equal intensity. They are at the receiving end of the disease as much as their loved ones.

Transcendental meditation endeavours to approach and address both groups. Equally relevant is the reminder that Alzheimer's, in its early stage, which we know as mild cognitive impairment (MCI), may not even be considered dementia. The subtle effects, involving either emotions or intellect or personalities, come into consideration years before dementia establishes its roots.

Transcendental meditation has enjoyed much publicity. In contrast to mindfulness meditation, in which distracting thoughts and feelings are not ignored but acknowledged and observed without any judgement, TM has a far simpler approach.

It essentially entails the repetition of a mantra for 15–20 minutes, twice a day, while keeping the eyes closed. Mantras are sounds or simple sentences that help the meditating person stay focussed. Attention is paid to overcome our constant outpouring of thoughts and to discover their source, which is felt as a moment of pure consciousness.

Simplicity and effortlessness emerge as hallmarks of this type of meditation. If we go back to a mind affected by mild cognitive impairment, we would appreciate that the undemanding approaches of TM that do not lean on an intact and superior intellect would be ideal refuges to adopt. In fact, the ideologies of TM endorse rather than resist the natural proclivity of the human mind to drift toward happiness.

The idea is that the wandering mind will find its way to happiness, drawn by the 'increasing charm' of its own blissful depths. The journey is a slow, smooth transition, from pure consciousness to a zone where one's awareness is suspended. With further practice, a permeation follows, allowing entrance into a space that is uncircumscribed and limitless, free from the shackles of thoughts, images or sensory objects.

TM and The Beatles

For decades, the easy-to-learn repetition of a few words during meditation sessions has captivated followers around the globe. The most famous were The Beatles. For all four—Paul McCartney, John Lennon, George Harrison and Ringo Starr—their time spent doing TM helped create moments of peace amid the vicious cycle of frenzied mobs, drugs and depression.

In an interview with host David Frost on a BBC show in 1967, both Lennon and Harrison talked of an elevated 'energy' that became their instant companions once they learned the techniques of TM.[1]

Frost asked, 'There were two things Maharishi [Mahesh Yogi]

---

[1]'John Lennon & George Harrison Interview on Frost Programme - 10/04/'67', *YouTube*, https://tinyurl.com/yyjxh6h5. Accessed on 7 December 2023.

said this morning that were the result of people meditating, following his system of meditation. The two things he claimed were serenity and energy. Have you found them?'

Lennon replied: 'The energy that I've found doing meditation, you know, has been there before—only that I could access it only during good days when everything was going well. With meditation, I find that it could well be pouring down rain, and it is still the same amount.'

Harrison had a similar answer: 'The energy is latently there every day, anyway. So, meditation is just a natural process of contacting it. By doing it each day, you give yourself a chance of contacting this energy and giving it to yourself a little more. Consequently, you're able to do whatever you normally do—just with a little bit more happiness, maybe.'

For McCartney, the effects were more profound and lasting. In an interview with director David Lynch, McCartney swore by its effects: 'I think it's always very good to get a sort of still moment in your day. Whenever I have a chance in a busy schedule, I'll do it, if I'm not rushing out the door with some crazy stuff to do. But yeah, I always like to take a moment and just meditate. Transcendental meditation is a good thing.'[2]

Following the lead of The Beatles, TM invaded all walks of our society, from business executives to teachers and students of all kinds. As one can surmise easily, the rapidity of its global influence hinges on a technique that is easily grasped and user-friendly.

TM for the Research Lovers

Therapeutically, TM matches mindfulness meditation trial by trial. Interestingly, results have come from the Division of Endocrinology and Molecular Medicine of the College of Medicine at the University of Kentucky. In 2007, a research

---

[2]'David Lynch interviews Paul McCartney about Meditation and Maharishi', *YouTube*, https://tinyurl.com/222aafdd. Accessed on 7 December 2023.

study team, led by primary investigator, Dr J.W. Anderson, revealed that the regular practice of TM strongly reduces blood pressure.[3]

Almost simultaneously, compelling results emerged from the Institute for Natural Medicine and Prevention at Maharishi International University in Fairfield, Iowa, showing decreased levels of cholesterol following the practice of TM.[4] Three years later, a study by the Perelman School of Medicine at the University of Pennsylvania demonstrated significant cerebral blood flow differences between long-term meditators and non-meditators.[5] Identical to what was seen in research involving mindfulness mediation, here too, with TM, scientists observed changes in long-term meditators in structures that underlay the attention network, as well as those relating to autonomic function, such as the heart rate, digestion and respiratory rate, as well as emotion. This is exactly why TM is emerging as a popular therapy to address the perils of a stressful life. Even short trials have generated positive effects. A mere eight-week meditation training study at Massachusetts General Hospital showed a significant decrease in activation in the right amygdala (a part of the brain important for emotions), supporting the hypothesis that meditation can improve emotional stability and response to stress.[6]

According to Dr Fred Davis, a leading neurologist and author of the book *Your Brain Is a River, Not a Rock*, TM erases that

---

[3]Anderson, James W., Chunxu Liu and Richard J. Kryscio, 'Blood Pressure Response to Transcendental Meditation: A Meta-Analysis', *American Journal of Hypertension*, Vol. 21, No. 3, 2008, pp. 310–6.

[4]'Institute for Natural Medicine and Prevention', *Maharishi International University*, https://tinyurl.com/2bepxa2d. Accessed on 5 December 2023.

[5]Newberg, A.B., et al., 'Cerebral Blood Flow Differences Between Long-Term Meditators and Non-Meditators', *Consciousness and Cognition*, Vol. 19, No. 4, 2010, pp. 899–905.

[6]Desbordes, Gaëlle, 'Effects of Mindful-Attention and Compassion Meditation Training on Amygdala Response to Emotional Stimuli in an Ordinary, Non-Meditative State', *Frontiers in Human Neuroscience*, Vol. 6, 2012, https://tinyurl.com/3hbv3bb8. Accessed on 18 December 2023.

line between challenge and stress, which means that one can take on increasingly more and more challenging things without it becoming stressful.[7]

Clint Eastwood, film actor and disciple of TM, had the same thoughts: 'I have been using it [TM] for almost 40 years now and I think it's a great tool for anyone to have, to be able to utilize as a tool for stress. Stress, of course, comes with almost every business.'[8]

The dance and dominance of meditation could not have been more timely. Studies conducted at the Department of Biostatistics at Johns Hopkins Bloomberg School of Public Health revealed that delaying the onset of Alzheimer's disease by only a year would yield nine million fewer cases by 2050. They also stated something more profound: that the prevention of dementia may be more effective with TM than with current drug treatments.[9]

CLINICAL APPLICATIONS: SUCCESS STORIES OF MY PATIENTS

Before I move on to mindfulness meditation, the other major form of inward contemplation, let me slip in two success stories involving my own patients, how they struggled, how they turned the tide and how they swam to their shores. But that's not the only reason I am highlighting these personal stories of success. I am also trying to emphasize that these successes did not come overnight. Holistic measures are not pills to be swallowed but procedures; and the results are not sharp bends of a boat but wide arcs of a ship trying to escape the iceberg.

---

[7]Davis, Fred, *Your Brain is a River, Not a Rock*, Create Space Independent Publishing Platform, 2012.

[8]'Clint Eastwood: TM is a Great Tool to Overcome Stress', *TM Blog*, https://tinyurl.com/499ej4v6. Accessed on 5 December 2023.

[9]Brookmeyer R., S. Gray and C. Kawas, 'Projections of Alzheimer's Disease in the United States and the Public Health Impact of Delaying Disease Onset', *American Journal of Public Health*, Vol. 88, No. 9, 1998, pp. 1337–42.

Mr Ricardo and TM

To my 80-year-old patient, Ronald Ricardo, it boiled down to 'just feeling god darn good'. Ronald had had his share of health issues, including diabetes, hypertension and high cholesterol. They were all under control because he regularly took his medications, but Ronald was unusually reticent during one of his visits to my office.

'Is everything okay with you, Mr Ricardo?'

No answer. Only a nod.

The physical examination was unremarkable except a heart rate that sped well over 100 beats per minute.

'You seem to be tense. Your heart is racing away.'

'I guess I am,' he whispered.

'What's bothering you, Ronald?'

'Nothing specific, Doctor. My belly hurts, my chest hurts. I am forgetting things like crazy. I am a mess...'

The last sentence was whispered with an exasperated undertone.

The story that came out was typical. His family-run restaurant had been on a steep downward slope. His grandson was on drugs. He had recently lost his sister, to whom he was very close. He was constantly forgetting where he kept his glasses and notebook. In short, he was stressed out.

Before I could address his plethora of ailments, he blurted out, 'But the last thing I want you to prescribe is lorazepam!'

I wasn't surprised by his answer, as I knew that Mr Ricardo would be the last person to find refuge in drugs.

'What are your thoughts on meditation?' I asked him softly.

'Way too complicated for me,' came his terse reply.

'What if it's way too simplistic by your standards?' I spoke.

Suddenly, he smiled. *What a relief*, I thought as he cleared his throat.

'What's on your mind, Doc? Time for you to talk.'

I explained the benefits of TM as a risk-free practice that was simple to follow. Ricardo agreed to a trial run and I provided him with the details of a nearby centre.

In the past three years, remarkable changes have happened in his life, despite the fact that his family restaurant is still struggling and his grandson is still a recovering addict.

'I am so much at peace,' he told me during his last visit.

Story of Roger Harper's Inward Journey

Roger Harper had a knack for numbers. As a corporate business executive, he had thrived on doing calculations in his head. But when he started struggling with familiar figures at the age of 63, he began to panic. His diminished abilities did not hit him overnight. At first, he thought it was the unending pressure of his job schedule and he took over-the-counter vitamins. The fumbling continued. Some days, he was fluent. Some days, he choked. Soon, he was stressing, which made matters even worse. Someone in his office mentioned Alzheimer's.

When Roger came into my office, he was adamant about not taking any medication. He had read up on the subject, and he knew there was no cure. I did the Mini Mental Status Examination (MMSE, a set of questionnaires to detect the mental agility of a brain) on him. He actually passed with a good-looking score of 26. I assured him that he was not harbouring Alzheimer's. I reminded him about the necessity of being knowledgeable and to be cautious about the vagaries of this disease. He prided himself on his intelligence, and I realized from his demeanour that he was deeply disturbed. He wanted the fumbling to be fixed. But the very fact that he was not in denial gave me the opportunity to propose an alternative approach.

'How about meditation?' I asked

I wasn't entirely surprised when Roger said he had heard about it before and had actually wanted to try it. He probably needed a physician like me to endorse the idea. I referred him to a certified instructor. For the past two years, Roger has been diligently practising meditation. He still works in the same firm, feels much more in charge of his numbers, and excitedly reports an overall poise and confidence he had never felt before.

THE BENEFITS OF POSITIVE EMOTIONS: STORY OF THE NUNS OF MINNESOTA

An extraordinary long-term study is being conducted since 1986 in Mankato, Minnesota. On Good Counsel Hill, the convent of the School Sisters of Notre Dame sits in tranquil grandeur. In what is popularly called the Nun Study, the Catholic nuns have offered their genes for scientific analysis. They have been tested on various subjects, such as how many words they can remember minutes after reading them on flashcards, how many animals they can name in a minute, and whether they can count coins correctly. Most importantly, they wrote autobiographical essays when they first took their vows. When the nuns die, their brains are removed and shipped to a laboratory where they are analysed.[10]

The brilliance of this ongoing study lies in the similarity of its subjects. The nuns have identical living habits, precluding any environmental differences. None of them smoke, drink or conceive. More importantly, they all eat the same food from the same cafeteria.

Published in *The Journal of Personality and Social Psychology*, an article about the study concluded that the nuns who expressed more positive emotions in their autobiographies lived significantly longer—in some cases, 10 years—than those expressing fewer positive emotions.[11]

Yet, inevitable questions arise: 'What exactly constitutes

---

[10]Snowdon, D.A., Nun Study, 'Healthy Aging and Dementia: Findings from the Nun Study', *Annals of Internal Medicine*, Vol. 139, No. 5, 2003, pp. 450–4.
[11]Danner, D.D., D.A. Snowdon and W.V. Friesen, 'Positive Emotions in Early Life and Longevity: Findings from the Nun Study', *Journal of Personality and Social Psychology*, Vol. 80, No. 5, 2001, pp. 804–13.

positive emotions?', 'Are merely positive emotions the main protective factor against dementia?'

We have already seen that a searching, intense mind does not guarantee safety from dementia. Dr Bharati Sharma, a brilliant obstetrician and gynaecologist, found herself drowned in abject dementia. Similarly, my grandmother, a scholar and a poet, wandered away and could not find her way back. Does the answer lie in a different direction entirely? We do not know the full truth yet. But it is becoming progressively apparent that stimulating mental challenges, such as solving crossword puzzles or reading tons of history books, do not necessarily prevent the onset of dementia.

MINDFULNESS MEDITATION: WHY PHYSICIANS FELL FOR IT

One of the most researched meditation techniques is based on the concept of mindfulness. Traditionally based on the Buddhist practice, it focusses on breath and physical awareness with a goal to perceive, without any judgement, the thoughts that clutter our minds. Mindfulness in particular allows a person to stay 'above' the tides of emotions that we feel every day. By conscious practice, your mind is trained to avoid falling into your usual, self-destructive behavioural patterns.

The ease with which mindfulness weds meditation reflects the profundity of the 'mindfulness meditation'. In order for the two words to be felt in unison, the two words need to be understood individually.

Very often, translation weakens the original word. Every monumental piece of work, every sublime slice of a short story suffers each time there is a change in the language. Be it Tagore, Maupassant or Tolstoy, that 'thing of beauty' fades a wee bit every time the primary source of expression is replaced. Yet, translation is the only way words can travel. Otherwise, Tagore would remain in Santiniketan, Maupassant in Tourville-sur-Arques and Tolstoy in the Tula province of Russia. To the translators of their works and others, we owe an unconditional salute.

The same credit applies to T.W. Rhys Davids. Born in England in 1843 as the eldest son of a Congregational clergyman from Wales, Davids studied Sanskrit under A.F. Stenzler, a distinguished scholar at the University of Bresla. As Professor of Pali at the University of London and founder of the Pali Text Society, Rhys Davids is credited as one of the first translators of early Buddhist texts.[12] The English word 'mindfulness' was coined by him. From the original Buddhist word '*sati*' was coined this giant of a word that, in the eyes of scores of scholars, has struggled to find the right home. Variously called or thought of as 'possessing a good memory', 'full of care', 'heedful', 'thoughtful' and 'being conscious or aware', 'mindfulness' was finally wrapped up in 2011 by *Oxford English Dictionary Online* as 'a mental state achieved by concentrating on the present moment'.

'*Smriti*', the word that closely follows the heels of sati, is another example of various versions of an ill-understood word running amuck. From remembrance, reminiscence and memory, this word, under the premises of the Sanskrit dictionary of Monier-Williams, is defined as 'calling to mind' or 'thinking of or upon'.

Caught amid sati and smriti, mindfulness at its very subtlest form falls in between a memory of the past and an attention to the present object of meditation in seamless continuity.

An Experimental Evidence

As expected, increased awareness from mindfulness meditation was quickly captured in a joint experiment conducted in 2007

---

[12]Guruge, Ananda W.P., *The Introduction to from the Living Fountains of Buddhism*, Ministry of Cultural affairs, Colombo, Sri Lanka, https://tinyurl.com/ysepjhts. Accessed on 7 December 2023.

by scientists from Oregon and China.[13] In this study, 80 healthy undergraduates at Dalian, without any training experience, participated. They were randomly assigned to an experimental or control group (40:40). Forty experimental subjects continuously attended integrative body-mind training (IBMT)—an ancient eastern contemplative tradition, involving body relaxation, mental imagery and mindfulness training—for five days with 20 minutes of training per day. Forty control subjects were given the same number and length of group sessions but received information about the relaxation of each body part from a compact disc.

A standardized computerized attention test measuring orienting, alerting and the ability to resolve conflict (executive attention) was conducted before and after the experiment. The results were equivocal and to the point: the experimental group showed significantly greater improvement in executive attention and alertness after five days of IBMT than the relaxation control group. They also reported lower levels of anxiety, depression, anger and fatigue, and high vigour when measured on the Profile of Mood States (POMS). Further, by measuring salivary cortisol levels, where IBMT participants showed significantly reduced levels, researchers logically inferred that stress levels were appreciably lower in the same group, compared to the control group.

But why select undergraduates? To my mind, this was a great scientific test. They wanted to obviate a possible bias that might creep in if the experiment involved senior citizens or devotees of mindfulness who were preconditioned to believe in the beneficial effects of meditation. A group of young men and women, devoid of these convictions and open to experimentation, was preferred and randomly selected.

---

[13]Xiaoqian, Ding, et al., 'Short-Term Meditation Modulates Brain Activity of Insight Evoked with Solution Cue', *Social Cognitive and Affective Neuroscience*, Vol. 10, No. 1, 2015, pp. 43–9.

EFFECTS OF MINDFULNESS MEDITATION ON UNITED STATES MARINE

Let us witness the effects of mindfulness meditation on US marines.

In 2014, Dr Amishi Jha from the Department of Psychology at the University of Miami, as well as Dr Elizabeth Stanley from the Walsh School of Foreign Service and Department of Government at Georgetown University, conducted a seminal study on active-duty military service members preparing for combat. In simplistic terms, mindfulness meditation training steadied the minds that tended to be distracted despite being on active duty.[14]

While this might sound more like an oxymoron, we can appreciate the subtle yet consequential difference between standing at attention, a body posture that conveys motionless alertness, and a mind 'at attention'. In simplistic terms, after years of rigorous physical training, not all combatants would have the same unwavering resilience and concentration of the mind as is witnessed in physical terms.

These assume immeasurable importance and potentially carry tremendous risks when we appreciate that these vocations require extreme situational alertness. It is a daunting task to address low probability events and fast-changing circumstances.

Unfortunately, these mind-wandering episodes are not exotic incidents to be dismissed as an exception to the law. Experience sampling studies have suggested that mental distraction despite being on a task takes place in 30–50 per cent of our waking hours.[15]

With that in mind, 80 healthy, active-duty US marine male volunteers were recruited to participate in the mindfulness-based mind fitness training component of this project. The entire training and subsequent trials were conducted at Schofield Barracks in

[14]Yeoman, Barry, 'Training the Brains of Warriors', *Mindful*, 3 July 2019, https://tinyurl.com/4cnr6kyp. Accessed on 5 December 2023.
[15]Ibid.

Hawaii, between eight to 10 months prior to the participants' deployment to Afghanistan.

While one group received an eight-hour and eight-week variant of the mindfulness-based mind fitness training, the second group received training that was essentially didactic, emphasizing stress management and resilience. The third group acted as a control, with none of the prior interventions offered.

A Sustained Attention to Response Task (SART) performance was assigned to all participants. The results unequivocally showed that compared to the no-training control group and those who only received the didactic course, the military cohorts who received mindfulness training had significantly fewer performance lapses.

THE QUINTESSENTIAL QUESTION: HOW CAN MINDFULNESS MEDITATION PREVENT ALZHEIMER'S?

Mindfulness meditation helps the failing mind in two primary ways. Alterations in brain nerve cells (neuroplasticity) and the brain waves caused by meditation offers a direct benefit in terms of better concentration, focus and memory. Mindfulness meditation also has a secondary effect because it decreases the risk factors that accelerate Alzheimer's. High blood pressure, high cholesterol, high cortisol levels, stress and obesity, all have been implicated in the establishment of full-blown Alzheimer's.

In a society where salt (sodium) is sprinkled on virtually every food we eat in fairly large doses, where stress has become a way of life, high blood pressure is a natural result. Intense interaction and collaboration between genes, environment, lifestyle and eating habits have brought hyperlipidemia and diabetes to the forefront. Not surprisingly, pharmaceutical companies have poured medications to combat these illnesses. Yet, true to the colours of a chemical compound, these medicines also offer side effects, drug interactions, and 'tolerance issues'.

The question one might have in mind is: 'Can meditation be

used as a complementary measure? Can it prevent or minimize our dependence on drugs?'

Strong evidence of its anti-hypertensive benefits was found in many research trials[16], showing that mindfulness meditation, along with yoga techniques, lowered the blood pressure of patients suffering from pre-hypertension, a state defined as blood pressure that is higher than normal but not high enough to require drug therapy. Pre-hypertension is associated not only with Alzheimer's but with a wide range of heart disease and other cardiovascular problems.

The 'active' group of patients undertook eight group sessions comprising body scan exercises, sitting meditation and yoga exercises for two-and-a-half hours per week. They were also encouraged to perform mindfulness exercises at home. The 'comparison' group received lifestyle advice plus a muscle-relaxation activity. The results showed that patients in the mindfulness-based intervention group had significant reductions in clinic-based blood pressure measurements.

Equally encouraging were the effects of Raja yoga meditation (a form of mindfulness meditation) on cholesterol, another risk factor for Alzheimer's.[17] In a study conducted at B.J. Medical College and Civil Hospital in India, 49 female patients were divided into non-meditators (those who had never done any kind of meditation), short-term meditators (meditating for six months to five years) and long-term meditators (meditating for more than five years). The results indicated that both serum cholesterol and low-density lipoprotein-cholesterol were significantly lowered in both short- and long-term meditators as compared

---

[16]Ponte, Márquez P.H., et al., 'Benefits of Mindfulness Meditation in Reducing Blood Pressure and Stress in Patients with Arterial Hypertension', *Journal of Human Hypertension*, Vol. 33, No. 3, 2019, pp. 237–47.

[17]Vyas R., Kanti V. Raval and Nirupama Dikshit, 'Effect of Raja Yoga Meditation on the Lipid Profile of Post-Menopausal Women', *Indian Journal of Physiology and Pharmacology*, Vol. 52, No. 4, 2008, pp. 420–4.

to non-meditators, especially in post-menopausal women.

As a precursor to Alzheimer's, stroke, coronary artery diseases, diabetes, high blood pressure and obesity has truly been the scourge of our society. While anti-obesity pills, weight-reducing surgery and nutritional supplements have taken centre stage, meditation has emerged as a strong, risk-free option to reduce body weight.

Stress, as we know, is virtually the epicentre of an ever-brewing storm. This risk factor can be singled out as relentless, ruthless and unstoppable. Whether it occurs as a generalized anxiety disorder or as a consequence of trauma, stress has an obvious psychological connotation to it. Stress has impacts well beyond the psychiatric realm. It can even push the mind into dementia.

The effects of meditation on reducing stress have been conclusively proven in multiple trials. In one of the most extensive meta-analyses ever conducted, researchers from Johns Hopkins University sifted through nearly 19,000 meditation studies and 47 trials that met the criteria for well-designed studies. Published in the March 2014 issue of the *Journal of American Medical Association (JAMA)*, the findings clearly showed that mindfulness meditation eases psychological stresses, such as anxiety, depression and pain.[18]

MATTHIEU RICARD, THE HAPPIEST MAN ON EARTH

Let us to turn our attention to Matthieu Ricard, a French genetic scientist turned Buddhist monk. Son of French philosopher Jean-François Revel and artist Yahne Le Toumelin, Matthieu was born in France in 1946 and grew up among intellectual and artistic circles. Showing precocious intellect since boyhood, he earned a PhD in cell genetics at the renowned Institut Pasteur, under the

---

[18]Goyal, Madhav, et al., 'Meditation Programs for Psychological Stress and Well-Being: A Systematic Review and Meta-Analysis,' *JAMA Internal Medicine*, Vol. 174, No. 3, 2014, pp. 357–68.

Nobel Laureate Francois Jacob.[19]

When he was barely 20 and at the threshold of achieving a lot, Matthieu unexpectedly travelled across the continent to India to meet great spiritual masters from Tibet. This was not the only time people had traversed with effortless ease from deep-rooted science to deep-toned spirituality. Matthieu made that transition from the busy alleyways of Paris to the sublime ranges of the Himalayas, where he met up with and took refuge in the hearth of the Dalai Lama. Since 1989, he has been serving as the French interpreter for the Dalai Lama. He is an active member of the Mind and Life Institute, an organization dedicated to collaborative research between scientists and Buddhist scholars and meditators. He is engaged in research on the effect of mind training and meditation on the brain at various universities in the US and Europe.

Around the same time, another scientist was embarking on a similar journey outside the realm of mainstream research. As founder of University of Wisconsin's Waisman Center For Investigating Healthy Minds, Dr Richard J. Davidson was exploring the neural bases of emotion and emotional style and methods to promote human flourishing, including meditation and related contemplative practices.[20] Named as one of the 100 most influential people in the world by Time Magazine in 2006, his studies have encompassed persons of all ages, from birth to old age, including individuals with mood and anxiety disorders, autism, as well as expert meditation practitioners with tens of thousands of hours of experience. Taking full advantage of an era of rapidly advanced technology, Dr Davidson has used a wide range of methods, including different varieties of MRI,

---

[19]Feloni, Richard and Daniel Richards, 'The Buddhist Monk and Author Matthieu Ricard May be the World's "Happiest Man," According to Science', *Business Insider*, 23 December 2017, https://tinyurl.com/rdhc57dw. Accessed on 5 December 2023.

[20]*Centre for Healthy Minds: University of Wisconsin-Madison,* http://tinyurl.com/4stxe4p2. Accessed on 7 December 2023.

positron emission tomography, electroencephalography, and modern genetic and epigenetic methods to see the benefits of meditation.

It was not at all surprising that Matthieu Ricard would fall under the radar of Richard Davidson. As a part of research on hundreds of advanced practitioners of meditation, Dr Davidson wired up the monk's skull with 256 sensors at the University of Wisconsin.

The scan results were breathtaking. Ricard's brain, when meditating on compassionate and kind thoughts, produced a level of gamma waves—that were those linked to consciousness, attention, learning and memory never reported before in neuroscience literature.

The scans also showed excessive activity in his brain's left prefrontal cortex compared to its right counterpart, which researchers believed gave Ricard an abnormally large capacity for happiness and a reduced propensity towards negativity. Research into this phenomenon is still in its infancy and Ricard and other leading scientists have been at the forefront of groundbreaking experiments across the world—an experiment or a series of experiments that embraced both ends of our planet, a bunch of meditating monks periodically journeying from Tibet to Wisconsin, inside Richard Davidson's Waisman Laboratory for Brain Imaging and Behavior in Wisconsin.[21]

We will examine what the researchers found.

The outcome was not just overwhelming. To the scientists, it must have felt like they were discovering life on another planet. Research from this unusual sample suggested that over the course of meditating for tens of thousands of hours, long-term practitioners actually altered the structure and function of their brains. They clearly demonstrated activation in multiple

---

[21]'Research of Richard Davidson Shows How Meditation Changes the Mind', *Waisman Center*, 25 June 2007, https://tinyurl.com/4nfph7a3. Accessed on 5 December 2023.

regions of the brain involved in monitoring, engaging attention and orientation.[22]

The results were fascinating. Compared to novices, those who did extensive meditation training required minimal effort to sustain focus. They also found that advanced levels of concentration are associated with a significant decrease in emotionally reactive behaviours that are incompatible with stable concentration, and that attention as a trainable skill could be enhanced through the mental practice of meditation. The reports must have shaken the scientific fraternity. Studies and trials poured in from all corners of the globe.

'We have been looking for 12 years at the effect of short- and long-term mind-training through meditation on attention, compassion, and emotional balance,' Matthieu said. 'We've found remarkable results with long-term practitioners who did 50,000 rounds of meditation, but also with three weeks of twenty minutes a day, which of course is more applicable to our modern times.'[23]

From all these institutional findings emerges one gracious fact we all need to know. Those areas of the brain that play significant roles in harnessing concentration, attention and focus are the ones that receive the most comprehensive benefit from meditation. In short, to prevent the brain from sinking into dementia, meditation is probably the surest and safest path to walk.

American neuroscientist Dr Andrew Newberg took the next step. Through sophisticated imaging studies, he could highlight increased flow of blood in meditators (and hence more activity) in the areas of the brain responsible for language, orientation and memory.[24]

---

[22]Ibid.

[23]'7 Meditation Tips From The World's Happiest Man', *The Way of Meditation Blog*, 29 April 2015, https://tinyurl.com/2t99ef7b. Accessed on 8 December 2023.

[24]Newberg, A., et al., 'The Measurement of Regional Cerebral Blood Flow During the Complex Cognitive Task of Meditation: A Preliminary SPECT Study', *Psychiatry Research: Neuroimaging*, Vol. 106, No. 2, 2010, pp. 113–122.

MY TRYST WITH WALTER FREEMAN: THE BEGINNING OF MY AUDACIOUS JOURNEY

We have flooded ourselves with facts and figures, straining to prove how meditation shines under the microscope. Yet, we know that objective results can take the pursuit of truth only so far. We also know that over and above these facts and figures are areas, uncharted but evolving beyond the laboratory but within the premises of a seeking mind, hinging on a willingness to trespass. For the sake of truth, we experiment. Yet, a greater truth eludes the experimental mind.

My first meeting with Dr Walter Jackson Freeman III took place in October 1999, under a cloudy Brooklyn sky on the premises of Long Island University. He was then a semi-retired theoretical neuroscientist, biologist and philosopher who worked in the labs of the University of California at Berkeley, pioneering research in how brains generate meaning. I was humbled by his aura of wisdom that instantly and happily humbled this onlooker. He smiled away most of my audacious inquiries as if they were bottles of moonlight. The ones that he chose to respond to were pure honey.

Later, as we ambled away from campus and settled down in a nearby Thai restaurant, we discussed his work. Among all his legendary works on chaotic dynamics, his writings on the fundamental aspects of happiness had pounced on me like one bright kid—attractive, willing and decidedly daring. Misquoted, misjudged, misunderstood and misled, the hunger for happiness has been the source of endless misery. Our conversations drifted to mind and memory, and this time it was his turn to plunge in with the typical childlike eagerness of a visionary.

Dr Freeman talked to me about his landmark article 'Consciousness, Intentionality, and Causality'. In it, he had defined consciousness as 'a global internal state variable composed of a sequence of momentary states of awareness'.

According to Dr Freeman, global state variable involves

'sensations, images, feelings, thoughts and beliefs' that 'constitute the experience of causation'.

'Do these make sense to you?' he asked me good-humouredly.

Of course, it did. In fact, I was happily surprised at how close it came to the definitions and viewpoints of what had been felt and preached in the ancient past. Consciousness, or what is called citta in Sanskrit, has being viewed as having the potential to know and think. *Citta* has no matter, no tangible form, or any place in which to remain. It is continuously changing.

To switch back to Dr Freeman's views, the brain evolves in a back-and-forth process of our reacting to sensations and images with feelings, thoughts and beliefs. Call it consciousness, soul or spirit, the attributes pertaining to the mind depend on one's *own* journey.

This conclusion takes on tremendous importance when considering the art of meditation. Unlike a pharmaceutical drug, which is swallowed with little personal initiative, meditation is an individual process that requires one's own motivation and commitment. You are challenging your mind, and thus repairing it in the process.

Powerful questions beckon us: 'How honest are we in our scientific pursuits? What forms the nucleus of such explorations—service to humanity or acquisition of power? Can spirituality help science?'

Fanaticism, be it religious or scientific, has forever troubled the world. The peaks and pinnacles of glorious discoveries have not been able to cure the mud and mire of our greed and bigotry.

CAN COSMIC POWER OF MEDITATION PRESERVE OUR CONSCIOUSNESS: MY NEW HYPOTHESIS

An event of paramount significance emerged from Freeman's concepts. He had often quoted British mathematician Sir Roger

Penrose, who in his 1994 book titled *The Emperor's New Mind* argued that known laws of physics are inadequate to explain the phenomenon of consciousness. He based this on claims that consciousness transcends formal logic. He took refuge in the principles of quantum theory as an alternative process through which consciousness could arise.

In a grand coincidence, thousands of miles away across the Atlantic Ocean, anaesthesiologist and the University of Arizona professor Stuart Hameroff was investing all his intellectual and creative energies on the essences of microtubules, (our vital cytoskeleton components) that he believed could be the cradle of our information processing system. He reasoned that the mystery of consciousness might lie in understanding these microtubules in brain cells, functioning at both the molecular and supramolecular levels.

The two were destined to meet and did so in 1992. What followed was magical. Hameroff lent his microtubules to Penrose's quantum theory. For the next two years, they researched the premise that consciousness is the result of the presence of quantum vibrations in infinitely small structures of the central nervous system, called microtubules. At a fundamental level, this meant that consciousness was derived from deeper-level, finer-scaled quantum activities inside cells, most prevalent in the neurons.

They both questioned the age-old theory that consciousness evolved from complex, mechanical computations among brain nerves. They argued the inherent omnipresence of consciousness as felt and preached by Eastern spiritual approaches for centuries.[25]

Suddenly, the terrifying path of amyloid plaques of an Alzheimer's dementia, targeting and wrecking these very microtubules, revealed an escape route.

Suddenly, I found myself asking: 'Can meditation, with its

[25]Penrose, Roger, and Martin Gardner, *The Emperor's New Mind: Concerning Computers, Minds, and the Laws of Physics*, Oxford University Press, 2002.

potential for neuroplasticity (alterations of nerve cells), replenish the dwindling quantum energy of the microtubules plagued by the onset of Alzheimer's?' 'Can meditation prevent degeneration, with its boundless capability to crystallize energy, before Alzheimer's arrives?' 'Can meditative electrical waves be preserved in the microtubules?' Suddenly, I am stumbling into a new set of hypotheses, incredible and enticing.

The possibilities are endless. We have seen this process before. Ancient sages advocated practices that rigorous scientific studies later found immeasurably beneficial. Monks lived in an age when nerve endings, let alone microtubules, were unknown. Yet, the calm and increased focus of sitting alone and concentrating for long periods produced results that performed better than any laboratory-produced compound.

BREATHING AND OTHER TECHNIQUES TO TAKE CARE OF YOUR HEALTH

It's been more than 30 years since I first encountered meditation as a boy. Yet, despite the ensuing years of heat and dust, those moments remain crystal clear, resonating with star-like clarity under a dark-blue sky.

As a young lad of barely 10, walking three miles was like crossing the street. My journey from home to the temple where I practised meditation was a 30-minute affair, something that I happily indulged in. The sun would invariably retire by the time I entered the entrance of the Golpark Institute of Culture, lodged in perfect serenity amid the swirling traffic of South Kolkata.

I loved to meditate. One could almost feel the chaos of a bustling city hungering for a spot of silence. But that was not the real reason. In India, meditation is practically a sport, a passion like soccer, basketball, cricket and other forms of entertainment. Every god sits in the meditative pose. Meditation is taught in school, cultured in scholarly circles and endorsed by health professionals. It cuts across state borders, religious proclivities and political ideologies. It is India's one solitary baton that is naturally and ceaselessly passed along.

Even today, my back can feel the soft, padded palm of the monk. That was the first step of meditation I was taught—to sit straight, with an unbent spine that would ceaselessly connect the sacrum to the atlas.

'This will create the right platform for the right type of breathing.' The monk spoke almost in an undertone as he straightened the thoracic curve of my spine. Years later, as a medical student, I learned the outstanding benefits of sitting straight. Slouching may not give a person a hunchback overnight. But if slouched every day on weak, sagging muscles, the whole skeletal framework can change. Much later in my clinical days, I realized chronic low-back pain is an inevitable outcome of a slouched and bent spine.

HEALTH BENEFITS FROM THE RIGHT POSTURE, THE RIGHT TIMINGS

So, what is a perfect posture? A perfect posture is one that is relaxed and straight, with a core of strong shoulder blades active but not tight, with an erect spine.

How does it help? The physiological benefits are immediate. A perfect posture expands the chest and enables us to take in a larger breath—a large gush of oxygen, vital for the lungs, heart and all our organs.

Before we attempt to unravel the basic building blocks of meditation, we must ask ourselves a fundamental question: 'What is the best time to meditate? Or is there an appropriate moment to meditate?'

To the retired and the relaxed, this is hardly a challenging question. To the working parent or college student, however, this can be impossible to answer—and even worse for the doctor who is working alternate day and night shifts. Ideally, from the spiritual point of view—and scientifically, too—moments of complete tranquility are most conducive. In meditation, we are talking about attention, perception and concentration—open or focussed. Silence is the language you want to hear. Globally, and across all religions, one would choose the crack of dawn, a time of enchantment only nature provides.

But how about the college student, studying late hours and sleeping like a baby in the wee hours of the morning? How about the nurse, exhausted after a long night of uninterrupted care and service? The solution lies in finding silence—anytime and anywhere, away from the screams of the outside world, in a comfortable corner.

When it comes to TM, the entire process of internalization rests on the mantra, the sound or word that is repeatedly uttered. Every religious being will attest that there exists a key word or phrase in their religion that generates tremendous power—be it in faith or in fervour.

HOW AND WHY PRANAYAMA ENTICED HARVARD UNIVERSITY

The technical intricacies of the practices of meditation and yoga are best left to certified teachers and seasoned practitioners. However, basic postures and breath control have weathered the test of time and emerged as fundamentals to be mastered in one's own space with relative comfort and ease. Western medicine pounced on it, realizing its magical combination of powerful effects from simple techniques.

It is relevant and prudent to mention here that *pranayama* at its deepest level is more than an exercise. In the spiritual context, it is not just a procedure of breathing in and out. The technique dives deeper into the subconscious.

For the purpose of clarity and accessibility, we will thus revert to the building blocks of breath control and take a brief sojourn into the anatomy, physiology and mechanics of our breathing. In most cases, they are intricately entwined.

As a combination of inspiration and expiration, the one structure that plays a pivotal role in the act of respiration is the diaphragm. When it contracts, it travels downward and, being attached to the lower ribs, rotates them towards the horizontal plane. The intercostal muscles attached to the ribs also contract and join the dance. The inevitable result is an expansion of the chest cavity. Fresh air, brimming with oxygen, gushes in along the branching airways into the fundamental air pockets of the lungs, called alveoli, until the alveolar pressure stands equal to the pressure at the airway opening. In perfect synchrony, blood enters the lungs through the pulmonary artery, picks up the oxygen, and starts its triumphant course through our body, blessing cell after cell with its basic cry for life.

The reverse happens simultaneously as, sapped of all oxygen and energy, blood returns to the lungs, carrying the toxic carbon dioxide that will be exhaled by a thoracic cavity shrunken by the relaxing diaphragm and the intercostal muscles.

What adds to this majestic display is the observation that the movement of the diaphragm is not a fixed act. In normal, quiet breathing, it moves downward for about 1 cm, yet on forced inspiration and expiration, its total back-and-forth could add up to 10 cm. This assumes tremendous importance when deeper breathing is solicited, either in duress or by choice. Unlike other body systems, the act of breathing is both autonomic and voluntary.

To the regular practitioner, striving for control of their own breathing, these become indispensable tools to exploit. It is a gracious fact that the controlling powers of the mechanics of breathing lie in the brain, where the respiratory centre in the brain stem directs the respiratory muscles. The medulla, located not far from the spinal cord, signals the spinal cord to maintain breathing, while the pons, a part of the brain located quite close to the medulla, provides further smoothing of the respiration pattern. The entire process is constant, continuous and completely involuntary.

Whether one is singing, playing the saxophone or simply verbalizing contempt, the voluntary part of breathing modifies accordingly. This sets the template of pranayama. The masters of this art control this very voluntary aspect of breathing. The word '*prana*' from pranayama has been frequently referred to as energy or 'life force'. This makes sense when we consider that the basic metabolism in our cells is an oxygen-dependent energy process. As researchers Ravinder Jerath and his colleagues working at the Augusta Women Center in Georgia learnt, the basic physiological responses from pranayama range from the cellular to the electrical. They proposed that voluntary, slow, deep breathing, as pursued in pranayama, functionally resets the autonomic nervous system and drags it away from its excitatory (sympathetic) state.[26]

In another landmark study, Dr Vivek Sharma and his colleagues from the Department of Psychology at Jawaharlal Institute of Postgraduate Medical Education in India embarked on an ambitious research to demonstrate the effects of various types of pranayama breathing techniques on stress and other cardiovascular parameters.[27]

Ninety individuals of both genders, all between 18 and 26 years of age, were drafted into the study. They were randomly allocated into three groups. Under the supervision of a certified yoga trainer, Group One was trained in fast pranayama (a six-minute cycle of three specific types of pranayama, with three cycles lasting one session); Group Two received slow pranayama training (a seven-minute cycle of specific pranayama techniques, with seven cycles lasting one session) and Group

---

[26]Jerath, Ravindra, M.W. Crawford and V.S. Barnes, 'A Unified 3D Default Space Consciousness Model Combining Neurological and Physiological Processes that Underlie Conscious Experience', *Frontiers in Psychology*, Vol. 6, 2015, p. 1204.

[27]Sharma, Vivek Kumar, et al., 'Effect of Fast and Slow Pranayama on Perceived Stress and Cardiovascular Parameters in Young Health-Care Students', *International Journal of J Yoga*, Vol. 6, No. 2, 2013, pp. 104–10.

Three acted as controls.

The entire study lasted 12 weeks and measured among others the major parameters of heart rate, systolic and diastolic blood pressure. Using Perceived Stress Scale (PSS) system, researchers measured the degree of stress perceived for all the three groups. The triumphant course of PSS has traversed well beyond merely tabulated reactions. Its implications have included objective biological markers of stress and increased risk for disease among persons with higher perceived stress levels. For example, those with higher scores (suggestive of chronic stress) on the PSS fare worse on biological markers of ageing, steroid levels, depression, infectious disease and wound healing.

The results were fascinating. All three parameters of heart rate, blood pressure and perceived stress were found to be significantly less in the pranayama groups. Not surprisingly, Harvard University wasted no time to adopt the fundamentals of pranayama.

HARVARD UNIVERSITY BREATHING TECHNIQUE FOR STRESS RELEASE

Let us finally climb down from the research savvy ladders and put our boots on the ground. What do all these research evidence mean in our practical lives? A look into Harvard University's hugely popular breathing programmes will show how seamlessly and successfully research trials based on ancient practices have transitioned to pure clinical benefits. Based on pranayama, a 4-7-8 breathing exercise has been successfully used for various sleep and cognitive disorders, including Alzheimer's. The technique is user-friendly and free of any risks. Let us get into the details.

Following are the steps:

- Lie on your back on a flat surface (or in bed) with knees bent. A pillow can be used under the head or knees, if that's more comfortable.

- Place one hand on upper chest and the other on the belly, just below the rib cage.
- Breathe in slowly through nose on a count of four, letting the air in deeply, towards lower belly. The hand on the chest should remain still, while the one on the belly should rise.
- Then hold your breath for seven seconds.
- Tighten the abdominal muscles and let them fall inward after exhaling through pursed lips on a count of eight. The hand on the belly should move down to its original position.
- It can also be practised while sitting on a chair, with knees bent and shoulders, head and neck relaxed.

Practice for five to 10 minutes, several times a day if possible.[28]

POWER OF SIMPLICITY: TWO MEDITATORS FROM ASSYRIAN AND JEWISH LINEAGE

I will end this chapter with emphasis and conviction on the preventive power of the word 'simplicity'. To that end, why am I writing about two disconnected individuals from two disconnected lineages? It is partially because I personally know and admire these meditators. But more so because they both demonstrate extraordinary simplicity in their pursuit of happiness. In a world of ceaseless clutter and clamour, their way of life stands out like a ray of light, soft, lambent, almost apologetic, yet promising and inviting, like an encircling embrace.

Nearly four decades of medical affiliation has taught me to value simplicity in every aspect of patient care. Be it as a physician, or a caregiver, or a nurse or a therapist, hallmark of any profound care lies in its simplistic attitude. The most complicated physical

---

[28]Ibid.

challenge or the deepest emotional suffering can be ameliorated best by a pair of simple hands, with or without gloves.

Every time I spoke with Shamash over the phone or met with Vasiliy in his little temple at New York's Brighton Beach area, I felt an exotic and exhilarating sense of simplicity, not just as an elusive human attribute but more as a liberating way of life. A release, a levity, a fine art that once mastered can unburden all that bogs us down, consciously and subconsciously.

I immediately knew as a doctor that this very simple trait is the drug of choice to overcome any stressful situation.

Shamash Aladina

According to Shamash, the power of simplicity is often the ultimate strength. Endowed with an emphasis on complete freedom and free from any tutorials, it revels in unchallenged supremacy. To him, this quality of simplicity seems to have come naturally. As a global teacher in mindfulness meditation based out of North London and the bestselling author of *Mindfulness for Dummies*, he has been instrumental in infusing peace and serenity to hundreds of people through his art of simplistic meditation.

To the stressed-out individual, fettered by frequent emotional and mental outbursts, Shamash's ways of meditation emerge as instantly possible, easy to grasp and enjoyable. To Shamash, any posture that is comfortable to that individual is a good posture. You could be in the traditional lotus pose or in more unorthodox positions, such as sitting on a chair, half-reclining with support on the back, or even lying down in a supine posture.

We might think that he is loosening basic ground rules of the game and compromising the results. On the contrary, I found great rationality in these relaxations. Comfort is essentially an individual experience. A person with back pain may find the spine-straight sitting posture more congenial than the half-reclined position. Similarly, the frequently short-of-breath asthmatic patient may find the half-reclined position more soothing than lying down.

An elderly person with an unstable gait would feel far more comfortable simply sitting in a chair with arms on both sides. One cannot aspire to mental peace from a body that is restrained, rigid and insecure.

As for breathing, the same simple singularity is adopted—a deep but unforced inhalation, followed by an equally relaxed exhalation. A 10–20 minute session can start as once a day and be extended to twice a day when one becomes more in tune with the practice.

To Shamash, the concept was more important than the technique. It was a concept where thoughts of both past and future needed to be released, again not forcibly but gently, almost lovingly. A tranquil, pleasant present is sought—a comforting present that welcomes all that is good and purposeful, despite shifting moods.

Shamash offered me a new word and I instantly lapped it up. *Kindfulness.*

It was as if the word 'mindfulness' had melted into the word 'kindfulness'. I realized this formed the very epitome of his approach. In the pursuit of mental tranquility, a certain benevolence is required for the mind that may have darkened with anxiety or aggression—an attitude that endeavours to be caring. And with it, comes a sense of acceptance of who you are, where you are and in what state of existence you find yourself. For once, I thought Shamash sounded like Reinhold Niebuhr, the American theological ethicist, who wrote in his 'Serenity' prayer:

> God grant me the serenity to accept the things I cannot change,
> Courage to change the things I can,
> And the wisdom to know the difference.

To Shamash, these become the attributes that need to be cultivated as one sits down to meditate. In what ways can one be mindful? Going by his approach, I was not expecting any complexities. Indeed, he kept it very simple.

One can be mindful of one's own body with a gentle, chronological tracking of one's own framework, from toe to the spinal cord to one's vortex. In short, this becomes a mindful sinking into the various layers of our body, system by system, organ by organ, possibly cell by cell. The same concept is applied to mindfulness breathing in the non-judgemental following of our respiration—the entire unforced process of spontaneous inspiration and expiration.

However, mindfulness does not have to be restricted to our bodily processes. It can be borrowed from nature. Sounds, natural and dulcet, can be allowed into and absorbed by the mind, just as thoughts or emotions. Emotions that comfort us offer peace and solace, and are equally compatible to a mind seeking tranquility, and so does the process of our quiet breathing.

Vasiliy Beniaminov

Vasiliy hails from Russia. Jewish by birth, Vasiliy was young and brash when he came across a Yogi named Aengar, in his hometown of Kislovodsk. Two aspects of that Yogi's teachings attracted him instantly: the flexibility of the dictums and the universality of the goals. There was an enormous temptation to seek freedom and happiness. Vasiliy decided to pursue meditation and yoga. Years of rigorous practice and discipline followed. He travelled to virtually all corners of India, seeking knowledge from all types of meditation and yoga. A follower of Lord Shiva, he is now called Siva, while his wife, going by Hindu mythology, is named Parvati.

Vasiliy is currently settled in the Brighton Beach area of Brooklyn, stretching from Sheepshead Bay to Sea Gate. Presently inhabited by Russian immigrants flooding the areas after the collapse of the Soviet Union and much before by Jewish survivors of the Holocaust, this ocean-encircling landscape is riddled with shops and apartments with a distance so litte that one can look into someone's bedroom from one's kitchen and hold elaborate conversations.

I met Vasiliy there when he was 65 years old but looking 20

years younger, both in structure and demeanour. He carried the same cherubic countenance I had witnessed in Shamash from England. He lit a candle and placed it in between us as we sat on our respective mats, face to face.

His English was halted and strained. Surprisingly, his words and phrases of wisdom came out easily. He spoke of all of us and of everything around us as 'reflections of our mind'. He was emphatic about science meeting spirituality to attain 'one single consciousness'. He went back to the preachings of the Veda to quote the five essential elements or *panchabhootas*: ether, air, fire, water and earth. When aligned with awareness, this is the avenue to achieving oneness. Vasiliy sounded relaxed all throughout, harboured a gentle smile all along and carried a refreshingly unrushed tone.

I requested him to show me some of the *asanas*. He obliged, willingly and happily, with minimal effort and with complete ease. He started with the pranayama and then moved on to others.

Vasiliy ended with the final pose of deep restoration after any yoga session—*shavasana*—derived from the Sanskrit word '*shava*', meaning corpse. It is essentially a corpse pose, where one lies down fully conscious and awake, yet completely relaxed.

Vasiliy practises meditation and yoga daily. He runs the boardwalk every morning, and holds lectures and workshops that draw in people from all walks of life.

'I don't remember being stressed out in my last 30 years,' he said. 'I am in good health. In fact, I have not been to a doctor in 20 years.'

SEVEN

WE NEED HEALERS, NOT JUST DOCTORS

'The wound is the place where the light enters.'

—Rumi, poet

DHRUBHA MAHARAJ: THE 'DOCTOR' I ALWAYS LOOKED UP TO

A scorching sun pummelled the near deserted streets of Calcutta. People retreated into buildings, shops, cinema halls, shades from any source to escape the sweltering heat. We were in a minivan. Myself and Dhruba Maharaj, a monk from the Ramakrishna Mission, were en route Sealdah to pick up saline bottles for patients admitted to Seva Pratishthan Hospital. The furnace-like milieu inside the van made sure we got drenched to the bone. I could have rinsed my handkerchief and squeezed out an ocean of sweat. However, what troubled me throughout the ride was not the uninhabitable, hellish conditions we were subjected to but the casual and almost callous smile of Dhruba Maharaj that hung onto his lips like an amulet.

I was a fourth-year medical student seeking hospital experience, and Maharaj was a resident monk in charge of the health division of that hospital. I later realized that there wasn't any mystery or enigma behind that smile. Maharaj was simply happy that he could finally sanction and secure such a large order of saline bottles. He had that smile on his face throughout the journey. On our way back, he would from time to time half turn and sweep his eyes across the bottles huddled together—tender yet firm glances of care, as if they were a cradle full of babies.

After reaching the hospital, as we walked between the rows of patient beds in the medical ward, I watched him caress one patient's forehead, take another's palm into his own, wave at another, all while harbouring the same lustrous smile.

At the time, I was still a good year and a half away from my graduation, and I wondered in what way was that monk less than an actual doctor? If the end point of any patient care is happiness and contentment, in what way was his contribution and commitment less than those who diagnosed and prescribed medicines? How much of patient care is treatment? And how much is healing? Do we know the difference between the two?

FATHER JOHN'S HEALING TOUCH

John Morley had a lively childhood in Boston, Massachusetts, where he blossomed into a successful professional with a master's in statistics and vast experience as a field analyst. The business world was his for the taking. But he was also having his share of earthly challenges. His mother had succumbed to a spate of chronic diseases, ranging from diabetes to heart disorders. Then came Alzheimer's, which bottled his father into a new, airless world of captivity.

One day, John's father wandered away from their current location in New Jersey. In genuine, predatory fashion, the disease devoured his sense of existence as he drove aimlessly for hundreds of miles during one moonless night. When he was finally rescued, he was somewhere in New York on Long Island. Unhindered, his health deteriorated in rapid strides. He was in a rush, as if to see the light at the end of the tunnel. He soon passed away.

John Morley found himself at a desolate crossroads, with an

abundance of challenges, which countless others have encountered. As a statistician, he could easily decode the predictable pieces of the puzzle. And then came a 'calling'. Amid the earthly darkness, he had a vision, infinitely more meaningful and deeper than the thin veneer that defined his earth. Becoming Father John, he strode out to his new, searching world.

As we sat in his cosy office, I learnt from Father John about his life, his philosophy and his mission. A table lamp lit two pictures hanging on the wall behind us. One showed Jesus with His flock of sheep and the other the smiling face of Mother Teresa. Both carried incredible nostalgia for me. The former took me to my convent school days. The latter was a personal remembrance that I treasure every second.

Father John has travelled far and wide, from Vatican City to Jerusalem. His intellect has ventured even further. From Christianity to Buddhism to simple humanism, he had let his mind follow the whole arc of his spiritual desires. He found a common thread in all these ways of life. Suddenly, he came to know his goal in life, his mission—*the path less travelled*—and he knew that it would make a difference. He would bring spiritual tranquility to men and women in emotional and physical distress. He would pray for them and *with* them, and together embark on a journey, however momentary, to find a land of eternal peace.

Standing 6 ft 2 in. tall, he was decked in a spotless black attire, with a pair of eyes almost pleading love and mercy, and a solemn smile forever hanging from his lips. Father John was as strong and as wanted as any life-saving treatment.

'Why did you choose to be in a hospital?' I asked, sensing his passion to be with distressed souls.

'What better way to serve God than through His creations?' he said gently. 'Patients appeal to me much more than any administrative work of a church.'

So, what is Father John's job description? To my deep dismay and deeper embarrassment, I realized I had little knowledge of his insurmountable contribution to patient well-being. My tunnelled views on inpatient care were stuck with intravenous and oral drugs, a plethora of lab and imaging investigations, and algebraic discussions with patients and their immediate family members. My rushed assumptions had thought of Father John as someone who was beckoned into a room filled with family members in a flood of tears, standing helplessly in front of a gasping body.

How then does Father John serve our hospital?

Truth be told, if there is anyone who spends more time with patients and their dear ones than any physicians, nurses and social workers, it has to be Father John—not in discussions, questions or giving verdicts; not in standing at the foot of the bed, mouthing diagnosis and prognosis but in interactions, intimate and soothing, seated at a patient's bedside, with compassionate hands, either folded in prayer or holding the nervous ones of others.

'Do you meditate?' I asked.

'Yes, when in deep prayer.'

'Does it help you?'

'Of course. You find a lot of peace, especially when in times of stress.'

I was at the Critical Care Unit one busy morning for a patient with congestive heart failure. Betty Ellmers was a frail woman in her mid-80s, whose past medical history read like a medical textbook. She had most of the major diseases one can imagine, including diabetes, hypertension and hyperlipidemia, and all their complications, including coronary artery disease, peripheral vascular disease and stroke.

This was not the first time Betty had been institutionalized. In fact, she had been under my supervision at least three times over the past four years. This time was no exception, except that she refused to interact. Her lips were sealed. There was no agitation, tantrum or crying spell, just taut silence. Betty was tired—tired of the cyclical, repetitive states of her existence. She was giving up on life and refused to budge from her adopted silence. Although she quickly responded to intravenous lasix, felt less dyspneic, and was soon out of bed in a chair, she remained nonchalant and unmoved by her progress.

That morning, as I was about to enter her room, I saw Father John inside. Betty and he were seated, holding hands. They seemed to be in prayer. I stepped back to give them their privacy. When I returned to Betty's room, she was lying on her bed. I wished her good morning. She did not reply. Instead, she smiled back—a luxurious full-teeth smile that reminded me of how she looked five years earlier.

WHY INDIA NEEDS HEALERS: SEEKING AN OPEN MIND

Allow me to write, as an open disclaimer, that by spirituality, I am not referring to religious proclivities, wrapped in rituals. To me, spirituality as an inward contemplation is an opportunity to think of life from a different stage, at once elevated and exclusive. In a hospital or in a nursing home, that opportunity becomes a necessity. Confined to a steel bed, a vulnerable set of eyes would look at me every time I would ask the traditional question to my patients, 'How are you?'

A sudden disorder, a slight sway from the norm, a physical or an emotional chink in the order… and instantly a new terminology arrives. A person becomes a patient. The comfort of a home bed turns cold and steely with potential rails. Comfortable custom-made bed clothes get dropped into one-fit-all gowns loosely tied at the back. Suddenly, one is enveloped by a new set of eyes, a new set of voices, a new set of professional tones.

Suddenly, doctors become gods, nurses become angels, therapists and other healthcare providers become guardians. One surrenders to new set of people with new set of tags—all professionally bound, all objectively oriented.

One wonders, where is the room for subjectivity? Where is

the room for life in times when disease and drug dominate? To put it more succinctly, when does a pair of gloves transition to a pair of palms gently touching the shoulder?

I have always believed that science has an opportunity to expand beyond its current boundaries if it embraces the eclectic ideas of spirituality. The individualistic aptitude of science pursuing the rationality of solitary parts of our system, be it our body or the universe, would stand in a brighter light if wedded with the holistic approach of examining the entirety of those very parts.

I am aware that I am treading into a battle-scarred field that has long cradled this endless feud between the upholders of objectivism and believers in subjectivism, each of whom have called the other counterproductive. Call it what you may, at the end of the day, this seeker-versus-pursuer conflict is still striving for one universal verdict—the truth.

It is refreshing to see researchers examine the effects of meditation and yoga through the latest technology we have, be it PET scans or MRIs. It is equally refreshing to see more meditators stepping forward to lend their brains to be probed and studied.

I am leery of terminologies. Alternative, complementary, integrative and mainstream are all medicines meant for the sufferer. An official Harvard Medical School definition of one of these terminologies runs as follows: 'Alternative medicine refers to those practices explicitly used for the purpose of medical intervention, health promotion, or disease prevention, which are not routinely taught at U.S. medical schools nor routinely underwritten by third-party payers within the existing U.S. health care system.'[1]

---

[1]Carleton, Jacqueline A., 'Broadening Horizons in Medical Theroy and Practice: Alternative, Complementary, or Integrative', *Body Psychotherapy Journal*, https://tinyurl.com/yut3zdu4. Accessed on 5 December 2023.

Why would you call a branch of medicine 'alternative' when more than 80 per cent of the global population uses it to their benefit? At a fundamental level, are not all of them essentially various options to be tried for the ease of suffering?

We must insist on valid options, as all of us know that there should be zero margin of error when it comes to addressing and managing human suffering. The process of validation, however, does not have to be identical. In their criticism of trials justifying holistic medicine, biostatisticians will point toward the Hawthorne Effect, a phenomenon in which experimental participants are influenced by the very knowledge that they are in a trial. They will also bring forth the fallibility of a perfect placebo in non-pharmacological trials. On top of that, the impossibility of achieving statistical significance without a double-blind study, where both participants and researchers are 'blinded' and made unaware of the options, are considered genuine reasons to dismiss such trials as a sham.

The brave healing step comes right from here. It is futile to hold the notion that the same trial design meant for a drug will be valid for subjective approaches, such as meditation or music. Just as bias-free results are tough to demonstrate in such subtle training exercises like meditation, drug resistance is equally impossible to be predicted in a six-month trial, especially when a drug can come out cleanly victorious only to stumble after years of use. These are necessary challenges that only reflect our own journey towards that truth we offer to suffering humans.

A clearer message emerges: A perfect trial may not necessarily lead to a perfect drug. Caught in the thick traffic of variable genes and changing environments, our biology is never etched in stone. Therefore, determinism—the process of simple derivations from conditions and laws—must have a democratic mindset.

Honest trials show the road to be taken, not a narrow, dead-end type of road, but one that is open to any number of lanes offering a way in or out.

CURE AND CARE

I first saw Mother Teresa when I was in sixth grade. I was returning from school one dusty late afternoon in June, an unforgiving month in Calcutta when the sun scorches the roads, even when the clock moves way past four. The bus had stopped at a red light and I noticed a group of nuns crowding around some bone-thin young boys and girls. A minivan marked 'Missionaries of Charity' stood at the corner.

'There's Mother Teresa!' someone said.

It was not hard to recognize her, as I had grown up seeing and reading about her in newspapers and other media outlets. 'Hearts to love and hands to serve' were her famous words for all.

Mother Teresa was known for her unconditional love and affection. With an unflinching faith in God, she revelled in selfless service to people in distress.

I saw her place her palm on the head of a young girl, whose unsure smile broke into an full grin, brimming with joy. An outpouring of tenderness followed, as Mother, not quite 5 ft tall and clad in a white sari with a blue border, leaned over and kissed the girl's forehead. I kept looking as long as I could, till the bus rolled away once the light turned green.

Since my childhood, I have tried to make sense of this relationship between cure and care. I always wondered why some volunteer with fervour while others remain unmoved and indifferent. Years later, as a third-year medical student, I posed this nagging question to Dhruba Maharaj. We were travelling together in a truck loaded with saline and dextrose bottles, to be transported to a nearby village clinic.

'What propels you to serve so relentlessly while you could have utilized your moments in the temple?' I asked, trying to fathom his feverish altruistic energy.

'Why I devote myself to service? Simply because I feel close to God every time I do.'

His entire tone had a rustic simplicity that was embarrassingly unpretentious. I had no response. It should come as no surprise that Father John too—from my present hospital affiliation— shares the exact thoughts and views.

As I proceeded through the years and tears of rigorous training, I felt a growing necessity to bring 'cure and care' together.

MY EXPERIENCES AT THE CALCUTTA RESCUE CLINIC

Like any medical graduate nearing the end of a training period, I walked a corridor of uncertainty as earthly matters took precedence above and beyond the hauteur of being a new MD. You either move into a clinical subspecialty, stay in your primary field, pursue private practice, or join nursing homes as a medical officer, who in an American set-up would be called a 'hospitalist'.

I instead opted for something that always attracted me each time I passed its venue. Calcutta Rescue Clinic functioned on the pavement of Middleton Row, a side road that broke away from Park Street, one of the most fashionable streets of Calcutta. At the far end of the street were two banyan trees, under which two makeshift tents were pitched. They were packed with medicines, syringes and files. The tents also carried boxes of bananas, apples and other breakfast items. Nurses and social workers huddled inside. All of this occupied three quarters of the pavement. The remaining quarter had a few stools where a few doctors could sit. Patients would kneel on street edges while the doctors would bend down to check their hearts and lungs. If they needed a chest X-ray or blood work, those would be ordered.

Treatment would be meted out beginning at six in the morning, when the entire scene would quickly come to look like a medical camp in a war-torn area, with hundreds of men, women and crying babies lining up along the street. These people would come from faraway villages, most sunk in abject poverty, with no access to any heathcare. Some would come barefoot and some wore sandals. Some suffered from leprosy or tuberculosis, while others harboured the usual quota of seasonal diseases. Patients would be attended in broad daylight for the next six to seven hours, occupying the entire pavement and half a street. They would be given tablets, injections and their wounds would be cleansed. By four in the afternoon, the camp would be cleaned up, miraculously vanishing. All that remained were the banyan trees, swaying happily over a spotless pavement.

All who came for treatment were offered a gift along with whatever medication they were given. Patients would be asked what was required and necessary in their daily lives. Accordingly, some received mosquito nets, bottled juices or blankets and quilts, while some got sandals.

I loved this approach, this ability to touch both the mind and the heart. While this hands-on, direct mode of a healing process was rustic and lacking in technological sophistication, its benefits were clear. If a society with a rickety, temporary camp can draw hundreds of barefooted, famished men, women and children every single day, then borders must be redrawn between what is appropriate and what is acceptable.

The heat and sweat notwithstanding, one of my most treasured and satisfying moments of patient practice took place under those tents, seated on sidewalk stools. All patients with leprosy and tuberculosis were diagnosed. Slick-skin tests and sputum and wound cultures were successfully conducted. Proper medications were given. No hurried assumptions were made. Even non-infectious, systemic disorders were diagnosed, referred to nearby government-run hospitals where they could be treated. Blood transfusions, stents and renal transplants were arranged. Follow-ups were performed with perfection. Intense and ethical patient care actually took place on a street pavement. We treated diseases and also healed patients.

FINDING OUR SOUL

I discussed these topics and many more with Dr Benjamin R. Doolittle during an annual scientific conference in American College of Physicians in 2016. Doolittle occupies a unique position in today's medical field as program director at Yale School of Medicine. He is also a church minister, so in many ways he is reminiscent of the good old days of medicine when a doctor could be a writer, philosopher and spiritual thinker.

Doolittle was lecturing on if, at the end of the day, we providers of cure and care had a soul. He was referring to physician burnout and if we had the coping mechanisms to handle complete mental, emotional and physical exhaustion. He was referring to a group of people whose profession was based on others' sicknesses, which is not always the most conducive of situations, considering the nobility and sanctity of the vocation.

How do we providers cope with internal challenges? According to a national survey[2] comprising physicians in training, venting did not work, Xanax certainly did not work, changing jobs made everything worse, and family pressures added to the woes.

What worked was a change of mindset, a practice of mindfulness and an ability to share. A perfect example is being on-call on Valentine's Day. It is a day fraught with thoroughly stressful conditions, when one is forced out of roses, restaurants and renewed pledges to the land of moans, groans and sighs.

Here is where a change of mindset is warranted. How about thanking the Lord for the opportunity to say Happy Valentine's Day to moaning, groaning and sighing patients? How about joining the families clustered in those rooms that lodge their loved one? How about replacing adversity with an opportunity for a different perspective?

---

[2]Patel, R.S., et al., 'A Review on Strategies to Manage Physician Burnout', *Cureus*, Vol. 11, No. 6, 2019, https://tinyurl.com/mztbt39r. Accessed on 18 December 2023,

Our minds and emotions can swing the pendulum either way. While the natural tendency to gravitate towards negativity tends to be the usual course, every chance exists to reverse the arc, be it through the unconditional faith that spirituality offers or through the optimism of a rational, positively-wired mind.

I once asked Dr Doolittle a direct question: 'Does spirituality make you a better physician?'

'What makes a better person?' he asked. 'Probably what makes me a better human is a good spinach salad, a gentle jog around the block, time with family, private time in prayer and meditation, and worship in church.'

Physics, as an indispensable branch of science, has crossed light years in its pursuit of answers. We have moved beyond Newtonian physics into quantum mechanics to explore areas of matter–energy duality. It has dared to address consciousness, rationalizing ancient concepts of a state that is neither material nor static. It is beyond a mere computable algorithm of a derivative process. In giddy delight, we learn from scientists that microtubules—those vital cytoskeletal elements and principal targets of Alzheimer's—are actually the primordial seats of our consciousness, huddled as quantum vibrations.

Dr Everett Koop, former surgeon general of the US President Ronald Reagan from 1982 to 1989, very aptly quoted the President, who once made a memorable remark while referring to his foreign policy approach: 'Trust, but verify!'[3]

This verification of trust is siphoning alternative medicine into mainstream patient care by blurring the borders and dissolving the frictions. Pharmaceutical drugs will continue to cure systems. Holistic measures will continue to reach the whole. The two together can heal the sufferer.

---

[3]Swaim, Barton, 'Opinion| "Trust, But Verify": An Untrustworthy Political Phrase', *The Washington Post*, 11 March 2016, https://tinyurl.com/38t7rx82. Accessed on 5 December 2023.

EIGHT

PREVENTION: THE FINEST ART OF MEDICINE

'Treatment without prevention is simply unsustainable.'

—Bill Gates, businessman, investor and philanthropist

I loved the Kelly couple. Married for nearly 50 years, both Dana and her husband Richard were childhood sweethearts. Standing at the threshold of everything that was possible and permissible, they had fallen in love the moment their eyes had met.

'Rich had the most powerful and elemental pair of eyes,' Dana hid nothing in her lavish praise. Richard had merely smiled and nodded, his face turning a tinge of crimson.

Theirs was a passionate love story. Dana nursed a strong Jewish lineage, while Richard came from a devoted catholic Christian family. Diana's goldsmith family travelled from the northeast post World War II to settle down in their prosperous diamond business, while Richard and his ancestors literally belonged to the Carolina soil, their plantation business dating from the days of slavery. Yet, neither the diverse businesses nor the varied ethnic or religious backgrounds stood any chance in the face of the fierce love of the teenagers.

Intelligent as they were, they bid time, created no unnecessary drama and quietly applied for the same college, the Ivy League Columbia University, which they both were desperate to join. And of course, fortune favoured the brave, as both Dana and Richard got accepted in their respective undergraduate programmes. Richard loved science. Philosophy was all that Dana doted upon. On a bright Sunday morning, they both took the flight from North Carolina for New York. They literally 'fled' the South.

As leaves of times fell gently over the years, Richard turned into a math wizard, teaching at the same famed university he had joined as a student. Dana joined a school at Upper West Side of Manhattan and eventually rose to the ranks of a no-nonsense, stern but a hugely respected principal.

When I first saw the Kelly couple, they were in their early 80s. An annoying upper respiratory infection resistant to preliminary antibiotics was troubling Richard. As I searched for a clue in his throat and lungs, ordered blood tests and sputum culture, I realized that there was more than a sore throat. His problems lay elsewhere. His words were minimum. The responses were tangential. Expressions were subdued. The constant smile hanging from his lips were not necessarily reflections of any happiness.

I performed a quick on-the-spot Mini Mental. Richard failed miserably with a score of 16 out of 30—way below the minimum requirement score of 24. I turned my attention to Dana, who was sitting quietly besides us, observing my questions to Richard with razor sharp eyes.

And then the pieces fell into their places. I had suspected what was going on the moment Richard had staggered into my room and wished me a 'Good Evening' while the clock had struck two in the afternoon.

For two years, Richard had been faltering with finances—an aspect that seemed ridiculous to Dana, as her husband was always the 'numbers' man. Her suspicion transitioned to fear when one evening she found an unsigned $5,000 cheque tucked in the pages of her recipe cookbook. That evening's fear turned into horror when she found out that her beloved husband, her object of all love and pride, had forgotten how to sign his own name. Sinking into gulfs of depression, then straining into fierce self-denial, the couple tried to beat the whiplash, holding on to things that were still undisturbed and carried on as if nothing had happened, as if the inability to sign was an odd happening to be dismissed; as if the occasional stutter and forgetfulness were a part of an ageing process, a necessary aberration, inevitable and hence to be trashed.

'But, why wait for two years?' I had asked Dana squarely.

She did not respond. But I knew the answer. A well-respected, dignified, graceful family could not accept any blemish in its otherwise unblemished sojourn. All this while, the clock ticked and Richard's dementia deepened, and an aberration turned into a ritual of unforced errors and tragic forgetfulness.

Many months later, when Richard got admitted with pneumonia, I entered into his room to find him aimlessly watching the ceiling. He failed to recognize me, his eyes wandering, nonchalant and meaningless. Dana, seated besides him, was deep in sleep, her hands firmly holding on to Richard's. I had no business to disturb their togetherness. As I tiptoed out of the room, I thought, what if Dana had summoned me two years before. Together, we could have at least delayed the inevitable.

PREVENTION: A WORD NON-EXISTENT IN MODERN MEDICINE

'Prevention' is an abandoned word in medicine—orphaned, disregarded and tossed to the side. I have always wondered why but could never come up with a plausible answer. Is it in our instinct to procrastinate? Is it our mindset that loves to indulge false hopes? Or is it just plain callousness and greed from those who control matters? It could be a rouleaux of all these, but the fact remains that Richard's mind, along with the millions of other minds and lives, could have been saved had they acted early. It is amazing how much scholarly, emotional and financial resources we have delivered since then and continue to deliver in the cure of human suffering, yet how little we invest in understanding and preventing the birth and development of a disease before it starts to brew and eventually cause damage.

Quite like the rest of the world, India cannot escape such a predicament. One of the pharmacy capitals of the world is also one of the epicentres of diabetes. How is this possible? How can a country with such powerful pharmaceutical industries, spinning out one anti-diabetic medication after another, be home to millions of diabetic patients? It does not need a genius to decipher. We belong to a culture where preventive measures do not exist. Conceptually, there is no awareness or education on the priceless benefits of dietary and lifestyle modifications. Same goes for high blood pressure or high cholesterol. The denouement is a circus of tragic events. Ungoverned and unbridled, these diseases run amok in our systems. As precursors and risk factors for heart attacks, strokes and kidney failures, they signal the inevitable. Pharmaceutical industries taste blood and generate pills. Doctors gleefully prescribe. Procedures are performed. A drugged society moves on, some falling by the way side, others trudging along. A perfect scene of imperfection.

Allow me thus, to focus on some omnipresent, objective and fundamental measures to prevent Alzheimer's from taking over our selves. Of all the measures mentioned in various sections of the book, I will highlight four of them as standout examples. None of them are guaranteed preventive measures but neither are they mere opinions. They are words of wisdom, tested by science and time.

Newton's First Law of Motion

Remember Isaac Newton's First Law of Motion? In simplified words, 'An object at rest remains at rest, and an object in motion remains in motion at constant speed and in a straight line unless acted on by an unbalanced force.' If we have to save our lives and live healthy, medicine needs to borrow the concept from this law.

Simply put, we need to be in motion, no matter what, how

and when. I have a catchphrase I never forget to tell my patients: Run; if you can't run, then jog; if you can't jog, then walk; if you can't walk, move your limbs; if you can't move your limbs, breathe! I go even further and advise, if you have a pair of eyes, then wink!

Bottom line is motion. What are we trying to move? We are helping in the circulation of blood and the oxygen needed by each and every cell of our body. Thus, be it the cells of the heart or the nerves of the brain, ample wash of blood and oxygen are the fundamentals of any cell's longevity.

Diet

There is ample research and evidence that shows that those foods considered healthy for the heart and the blood vessels are equally helpful for the brain.[1] Let us revisit them:

Green leafy vegetables: Our brain needs nutrients like vitamin K, lutein, folate and beta-carotene to preserve our sense of cognition. As sources of these invaluable nutrients, leafy greens such as kale, spinach, collards and broccoli are priceless.

Fatty fish: Fish replete with Omega-3 fatty acids have become our darlings after research showed that they reduce the brain damaging protein found in Alzheimer's-affected brain, the beta amyloid. Go for fish with low mercury, like salmon, cod, tuna and pollock. With high levels of Omega-3 fatty acids and moderate to low levels of mercury, Indian Rohu and Hilsa fish are thus equally acceptable.[2]

Berries: Blueberries carry a natural pigment called flavonoids

---

[1]'Foods Linked to Better Brainpower ', *Harvard Health Publishing*, 6 March 2021, https://tinyurl.com/2hftpsaf. Accessed on 8 December 2023.

[2]Canhada, S., et al., 'Omega-3 Fatty Acids' Supplementation in Alzheimer's Disease: A Systematic Review', *Nutritional Neuroscience*, Vol. 21, No, 8, 2018, pp. 529–38.

that are invaluable resources for memory preservation. One or two servings of these berries will always help our brain.

Caffeine: If you cannot start your day without *that* cup of coffee or tea, so be it! Caffeine has been proved to have strong mental preservation powers. But, of course, like everything else, intake should never transition to indulgence, for an excess causes acidity.[3]

Walnuts: An invaluable ingredient of the heart-healthy Mediterranean diet, containing alpha linolenic acid (ALA), a substance proved to have beneficial effects on our memory, walnuts are our best friends when it comes to the brain and heart.[4]

Being with Others and Yourself

Our discussion invariably turned to happiness and the necessity of bondage whenever and wherever I met Berkeley neuroscientist and philosopher Dr Walter Freeman. He would cite one of his articles 'Happiness Doesn't Come in Bottles'[5] to prove that socialization and bondage are the *prime de force* for maintaining the functional integrity of our brain. I always agreed with him, not just as a validation of his wisdom and intellect, but also through my near 40 years as a scientist and a physician who has observed, experienced and experimented on the indispensability of human interaction in maintaining cognitive function.[6] Nothing can be more brain-friendly than heart-warming sessions between children and their parents, grandchildren and their grandparents or just two souls laughing over a cup of tea.

---

[3]Borota, D., et al., 'Post-Study Caffeine Administration Enhances Memory Consolidation in Humans', *Nature Neuroscience,* Vol. 17, No. 2, 2014, pp. 201–3.
[4]Féart, Catherine, et al., 'Mediterranean Diet and Cognitive Function in Older Adults', *Current Opinion in Clinical Nutrition and Metabolic Care,* Vol. 13, No. 1, 2010, pp. 14–8.
[5]Freeman, Walter, 'Happiness Doesn't Come in Bottles', *Sisyphus,* https://tinyurl.com/3sdfmafs. Accessed on 8 December 2023.
[6]Sen, Shuvendu, 'Origin of Happiness – Biology or Beyond?', *The Times of India,* 26 November 2011, https://tinyurl.com/mw8cvtxs. Accessed on 8 December 2023.

As dealt in details in my previous chapters, some moments with oneself can also act as powerful allies for your brain health. Be it music, meditation or reading a novel, these inward journeys are necessary luxuries every brain cell will beseech. To not be lonely when alone, to seek one's own company in solitude, to write a love letter to oneself are actually strong practical exercises where philosophy melts into science.

The 'Big Five Personality Traits' and How Some of Them Can Prevent Dementia

Conceptualized by British scientist Sir Francis Galton in 1884 and subsequently developed and honed by leading psychologists from across the academic world, five major personality traits have been identified. But what has taken the scientific world by storm has been the recent realization that some of these traits if cultured and nurtured diligently can be used to protect us from Alzheimer's. To get to the crux of the study[7], it has been found that traits like conscientiousness (ability to be organized and efficient), agreeableness (being friendly and compassionate), extraversion (being outgoing and energetic) and openness to experience (being inventive and curious) have strong protective effects on our brain as opposed to neuroticism (being nervous and sensitive) and overall scepticism that seem to promote and provoke dementia.

IN ALZHEIMER'S, PREVENTION IS PRIMORDIAL

When it comes to healing Alzheimer's, we face the crisis whether scientists detect an exclusive pathology at its very inception? Can they diagnose the disease when only a hint exists? Along with

---

[7]Singh-Manoux, A, et al., 'Association of Big-5 Personality Traits with Cognitive Impairment and Dementia: A Longitudinal Study', *Journal of Epidemiology Community Health*, Vol. 74, No. 10, 2020, pp. 799–805.

our intellectual aggression to develop new cures, can we foster an equivalent fervour to capture the disease before it can mature? I certainly hope we can. But before that, we need to remove the rust that has collected in the arts of detection and diagnoses that once were considered masterpieces. We need to start all over again as students of truth, with the belief that permanence of any solution lies in the prevention of that very problem.

While we await the magic cure for Alzheimer's disease, let us prevent the inevitable. Let us arc back to our primordial organs, our eyes, our ears and our awakened minds. Let us together fight with all our resources and courage against a disease that can and must be conquered.

ACKNOWLEDGEMENTS

It is my absolute pleasure to acknowledge the contributions of many people in this book.

For any writer's flight, howsoever daring and delightful, a point of entry is a necessity. A point that crystallizes the inspired moments, governs the cruise, deepens the thoughts and eventually elevates an unsure manuscript to a solemn deliverance of substance. For these and many more, I owe deeply to Dibakar Ghosh, editorial director, Rupa Publications. From the title to the reference, every page of this book has his thumb of advice, stewardship and insight.

To him and to the entire team of Rupa Publications, from cover design to copy editing, I am deeply grateful to everyone. Special thanks to Sakschi Verma, the copy editor of this book, for her brilliant insights, intuitive thoughts and detailed guidance.

To Shiladitya Chaudhuri, one of the finest entrepreneurs I have come across in recent times, I owe my limitless debt for not only his vast harvest of resources that he provided but also for his courage that I unabashedly borrowed to deal with the improbable and the uncharted. To him and to his brilliant team from Sagittarius Communications, I remain indebted.

At the Optimal Media Solutions, Times Group, I have the pleasure of working with a team of talented and dedicated, brilliant professionals with Sumanta Chatterjee in the lead. Their publicity and networking talents are and will be the key to the nationwide spread of this book. Thank you, Sumanta.

My salute to all the authors across the world of medicine, whose pens have matched their skills and dexterity in the art of patient care. Indeed, to them and to all writers and scholars, I bow in gratitude for their immense influence and relentless guidance, not the least being my mother Sujata Sen who is and always will be my favourite author.

I also owe a special thanks to the extraordinary companionship I have been privileged to receive from Bob Roy, former Times Response editor (East), The Times of India Group, BCCL. A sounding board, Bob has always been the retreat of all my literary whims and wishes.

I owe my limitless gratitude to Aaron Feingold, MD, author, brilliant academician and chief of cardiology, JFK Hospital; Ronald Brenner, MD, founder, CEO and principal investigator of Neurobehavioral Research Inc.; and Andrew Newberg, MD, director of research, Marcus Institute of Integrative Health, Jefferson University Hospital for not only their unflinching support and endorsement in all my medica-literary endeavours but also for their limitless repertoire and repository of basic and applied medical knowledge.

To Chandana Mitra and Bidisha Sen, I extend my deepest respect for bravely coming forward to relate their own tales of emotional challenges concerning their parents.

And my deepest thanks to my family: my wife, Paramita Sen, for her unfailing faith in me as a person and a writer; my daughter and son, Brinda and Rik, for their unending and fierce support and fellowship; and my sisters and parents, for their support have been the light that guides me.

This book is incomplete without my undeterred gratitude and bow to my patients and their caregivers, whose indomitable and unputdownable courage will always remain the sustenance, source and inspiration of my writings and patient care.

INDEX